From Birth to Sixteen

From Birth to Sixteen outlines children's physical, social, emotional and linguistic development from infancy through to adolescence. In both its practical application of research and its contribution to the assessment of child development, this text provides essential reading for those studying, or indeed practising, child development in the context of nursing, play work, youth work, play therapy, early years education, teaching, social work and occupational therapy.

This innovative text is accessible and engaging, with case studies, tables and references to relevant studies making links to professional practice throughout. Designed to fit with the requirements of the Common Assessment Framework, it presents developmental models for the years from birth to sixteen under the following themes:

- children's rights and responsibilities
- relationships in the family
- relationships in day care, at school and with the peer group
- language and communication
- children and the media
- health issues in childhood and adolescence
- emotional well-being and resilience.

A dedicated companion website offers additional teaching and learning resources for students and lecturers, including an interactive timeline, further case studies and extensive self-assessment material.

Crucially, the text appreciates the diversity of ways in which children develop, taking into account gender, ethnicity, social background and disability, and it values children's resilience in conditions of adversity. From the foundations of the subject through to its application in practice, *From Birth to Sixteen* provides an indispensable companion to child development courses and beyond.

Helen Cowie is Professor Emeritus and Director of the UK Observatory for the Promotion of Non-Violence (www.ukobservatory.com) at the University of Surrey in the Faculty of Health and Medicine. A psychologist by background, she teaches a range of education, psychology, and health and social care students. For over 20 years she has specialized in strategies to counteract school bullying, including peer support as an effective intervention that empowers children and young people to take action themselves to help other young people who are experiencing social and emotional difficulties. Her widely-used training manual *Peer Support in Action*, co-authored with Patti Wallace, influenced practice in the UK and other European countries. In 2009 it was translated into Japanese following a long-standing collaboration with the Japanese Peer Support Association.

In *Managing School Violence*, she and co-author Dawn Jennifer designed training for a whole-school approach to reduce and prevent bullying, while *New Perspectives on Bullying* emphasized the importance of fostering positive relationships in the school community as a whole and provided a wealth of evidence-based good practice for professionals. Her co-authored book *Understanding Children's Development* remains one of the most popular undergraduate psychology textbooks in the field and a fifth edition was published in September 2011.

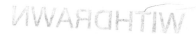

Reviews of *From Birth to Sixteen*

'A valuable and timely source of information on child development, from birth to sixteen. This text addresses key issues and theories in relation to the developing child in a clear and contemporary manner with enough detail to facilitate understanding of key concepts.'
Wendy Sims-Schouten, University of Portsmouth, UK

'This is an excellent book and a must for all practitioners working with children and young people. The author encompasses a wide range of relevant and sensitive issues in a thorough, practical and informed way. Not only is this text a sound contribution to our understanding of childhood from birth to sixteen but it is also a most enjoyable read.'
Sean MacBlain, University College Plymouth St Mark & St John, UK

'*From Birth to Sixteen* provides an excellent comprehensive coverage of the main areas affecting children and early teenagers. It explores key areas of development, emotional health, communication and behaviours and is an essential core text for both students and practitioners alike. The book successfully integrates theoretical and real world perspectives in an accessible and meaningful way. I would highly recommend this text for those studying issues affecting children.'
Will Medhurst, University of Portsmouth, UK

From Birth to Sixteen

Children's health, social, emotional and linguistic development

Helen Cowie

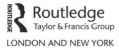

Routledge
Taylor & Francis Group

LONDON AND NEW YORK

First published 2012
by Routledge
2 Park Square, Milton Park, Abingdon, Oxon OX14 4RN

Simultaneously published in the USA and Canada
by Routledge
270 Madison Avenue, New York, NY 10016

Routledge is an imprint of the Taylor & Francis Group, an informa business

British Library Cataloguing in Publication Data
A catalogue record for this book is available from the British Library

Library of Congress Cataloging-in-Publication Data
Cowie, Helen.
From birth to sixteen : children's health, social, emotional and linguistic development / Helen Cowie.
p. ; cm.
Includes bibliographical references.
I. Title.
[DNLM: 1. Child Development. 2. Adolescent Development. 3. Emotions. 4. Personality Development. WS 105]
618.92–dc23
2011036383

ISBN 13: 978–0–415–60265–5 (hbk)
ISBN 13: 978–0–415–60266–2 (pbk)
ISBN 13: 978–0–203–12635–6 (ebk)

Typeset in Sabon and Frutiger by
Keystroke, Station Road, Codsall, Wolverhampton

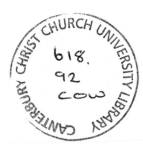

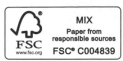

Printed and bound in Great Britain by
TJ International Ltd, Padstow, Cornwall

Dedicated to Corrie, Isabel and Haruki
(from birth to 14)

Contents

Preface

In writing *From Birth to Sixteen* I intended to create an evidence-based resource for all professionals who work with and care about children and young people. It seemed straightforward at the beginning simply to describe 'good enough' parenting and care as a model. What emerged in the process was an increasing awareness of the sheer diversity of young people's lives and the impossibility of capturing all aspects of their experience. On the one hand, it was important to document the main stages of typical development; on the other, it was essential to include, without being judgemental, the experiences of children and young people who, for whatever reason, had particular risk factors in their lives. It was important to demonstrate the resilience of vulnerable children and young people in the face of adversity without minimizing the responsibility of adults, communities and the wider society to provide the best opportunities for the next generation. It was necessary to be selective with regard to major health risks that face children and young people in today's society. It was not possible to include every disorder or disability within the text. However, the book covers substantial health risks that include obesity, eating disorders, addictions, unplanned pregnancy and abusive sexual behaviour, and mental health difficulties.

So, *From Birth to Sixteen* contains many examples of intervention programmes that aspire to prevent risks to social, emotional, language and health development as well as to strengthen protective factors within individuals, their families, communities and schools. My aim throughout the book has been to document the resilience within children and young people, the characteristics of their families and the characteristics of the wider social environment. Protective resources are necessary in each one of these contexts. I hope that *From Birth to Sixteen* succeeds in convincing the reader of the need to view the developing young person in their social and cultural context. I hope, too, to convince readers of the crucial importance of significant relationships with adults and peers for the young person's emotional development. These relationships lie at the heart of the child's development and must be nurtured and strengthened in every context in which the young person lives, learns, plays and socializes. All adults who work with young people must be aware of the need for sensitive attunement to their needs.

The text of *From Birth to Sixteen* is only one aspect of a much larger project. There is a companion website available online. A key feature is the interactive timeline for easy reference to major milestones that children and young people progress through with regard to social, emotional and language development. There is also information on children with special educational, behavioural and social needs. This website links to other helpful websites and provides a range of video clips and case studies to illustrate key aspects of development. There are also links to relevant research reports, government reports, NGO sites and key journal articles on significant research in this ever-expanding field. For students and instructors, there are resources including self-assessment and multiple-choice questions, chapter summaries, discussion topics, revision guides and small-scale tasks and investigations. It is planned that these will be regularly updated in the light of feedback from readers and I would be interested to hear from you.

I am indebted to the healthcare and education professionals and researchers who so generously shared their knowledge with me. Throughout the book I have made use of the experiences of children and young people through illustrative case studies in order to give greater depth to the concepts being discussed. It is my hope that these voices help the reader to understand more deeply the richness of the experiences documented in this way.

Helen Cowie

Acknowledgements

I would like to acknowledge the help and guidance offered by Martyn Barrett, Mark Blades, Pat Colliety, Anthony Daly, Gill Francis, Anita Green, Gill Haddock, Vavi Hillel and John Quirk, as well as the comments from a panel of anonymous reviewers.

Chapter 1

The developing child

There are complex interactions between socio-economic, health, educational and socio-emotional factors in any child's development. Children and young people are physically healthier in the twenty-first century than they were in the past and there are now many more professionals supporting families than ever before. In the twenty-first century, infant mortality rates in the UK are generally low, at less than 0.1% of the child population. This was not always the case. At the beginning of the nineteenth century, around 10% of children did not survive their first year of life. Among the poor, this rate was 20%. Causes of death included epidemics of measles, scarlet fever, whooping cough as well as poor nutrition, contaminated water and environmental factors such as low-standard housing.

Despite the advances in education, health and social care for children, there are still major concerns. There remain unacceptable health variations among different social groups in the UK. For example, based on data about children born in 2005, infant mortality in Pakistani and Caribbean groups was twice that of the White British groups. Babies born in Pakistani and Caribbean families had infant mortality rates of 6.9 and 7.8 deaths respectively per 1,000 live births in comparison with 4.2 deaths per 1,000 live births in the White British group (ONS, 2011a). In comparison with the majority White population, children in minority communities are more likely to experience disadvantage and discrimination, and to be living in poverty. According to Barnardo's (2007), 27% of White British children live in poverty compared with 48% Black and Black British and 67% Pakistani and Bangladeshi. Serious outcomes are that families living in poverty experience poorer health, have reduced life expectancy and, in some areas of the UK, have more difficulties in accessing health resources (Vydelingum & Colliety, 2011).

With regard to children's emotional health and well-being, there is strong evidence for an increase in psychosocial disorders during childhood and adolescence (Aynsley-Green, 2009; Rutter & Smith, 1995). The Innocenti Report published by UNICEF (2010) provided evidence that, in comparison with other countries in the developed world, children in the UK scored very poorly in terms of emotional health and well-being. The UNICEF study found that UK children rated their own health as being low, and they also described themselves as the least content in the developed world and as more likely to feel lonely and excluded. In comparison with other countries, children in the UK are more likely to have been drunk. Rates of under-age sex are high, as is the incidence of teenage pregnancy.

Emotional and behavioural difficulties among children and young people have increased over the past four decades (MHF, 1999; Rait et al., 2010). An international study of child well-being in the developed countries (UNICEF, 2007) reported that the UK ranked in the bottom third. The emotional health and well-being of children and young people has been highlighted by successive governments as an area of concern (DCSF, 2008; DH, 2004). Today's young people seem to face severe stresses that were unknown a generation ago. Suicidal thoughts are common among young people, as are feelings of hopelessness and futility; two-thirds of suicidal young men feel that they have no one to turn to for help (Samaritans, 2000). Certain groups of young people are especially vulnerable, including young carers, looked-after children, children of asylum seekers and children living in disadvantaged areas. For example, research carried out jointly by The Princess Royal Trust for Carers and The Children's Society (2011) found that a quarter of *young carers* – children or young people who are responsible for caring for an adult in their family who is ill – aged 6–18 years suffered stress because of juggling their family responsibilities and school work; they were also more likely to be bullied by peers at school. There are disturbing statistics on the number of children and young people who run away from home or care. A *runaway* is defined as a child or young person under the age of 16 who has spent one night or more away from home without parental permission. These amount to around 100,000 episodes each year in the UK, with around a quarter running away before the age of 13, and one in ten running away before the age of ten (ibid., 2011). While a child who has gone missing will be reported to the police, this is not the case for most runaways. Tragically, in most cases, these children and young people neither seek nor receive professional help, despite the fact that they are at high risk of physical abuse or sexual exploitation.

Current government policies aspire to achieve better health outcomes for children through provision of health, social and education services for all, and progress in minimizing health and educational inequalities. The infrastructure that contributes to continuing reductions in child death and illness includes policies for immunization against common childhood illnesses, systems for safe drinking water, safe food, improved housing conditions, better quality of air, road safety campaigns and wider knowledge about healthy eating and healthy lifestyles. Government policies provide a framework in which to deliver an array of services to meet the psychological as well as the physical needs of children and young people. These services are delivered through, for example, the *National Service Framework for Children, Young People and Maternity Services*, *The Children's Plan* and through the *Every Child Matters* agenda. Public health concerns regarding children and young people at present include as a priority the issues of obesity, mental health, social health and teenage pregnancy. The public health White Paper, *Healthy Lives, Healthy People* (DH, 2010), highlights sexual health as a key issue and proposes a new integrated sexual health policy, to include confidential, non-judgemental services on sexually transmitted infections (STI), contraception, abortion, health provision and advice on prevention. The UK committed itself to provide at least the minimum standards as stated in the UN *Convention on the Rights of the Child* (UN, 1989). For example, Article 19 states that all children have the right to be protected from physical and mental violence.

Despite this public concern, some children continue to be abused and neglected by their parents or carers and there is unequivocal evidence that this has extremely serious consequences for the child's development. At the time of writing, in the UK the National Society for the Prevention of Cruelty to Children (NSPCC) has some 30,000 cases of children on their child protection register, a rate of 0.25% of the population (NSPCC, www.nspcc.org.uk) and some writers suggest that the actual figure may be much higher. The outcomes are tragic. Around 200 UK children die each year as a result of direct or indirect abuse by their parents; child abuse is the fourth commonest cause of death in pre-school children. For those who survive, the outcomes include increased risk by the time of adolescence of depression, eating disorders, drug misuse and involvement in crime and violence. By adolescence, children who have been abused

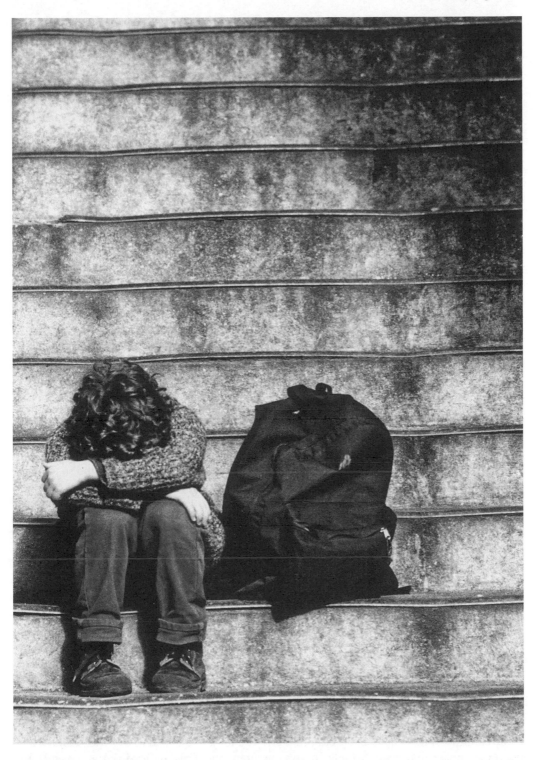

Getty images

or neglected by their parents are more likely to have relationship difficulties and, in their turn, to find the process of parenting a challenging experience.

The (UNICEF) Report Card series proposes that 'the true measure of a nation's standing is how well it attends to its children – their health and safety, their material security, their education and socialization, and their sense of being loved, valued and included in the families and societies into which they are born'. Its recurring theme is that 'protecting children during their vital, vulnerable years of growth is both the mark of a civilized society and the means of building a better future' (UNICEF, 2010: 1). With this precept in mind, *From Birth to Sixteen* aims to give knowledgeable support and information to all those who work with children and young people, and who wish to give them the best opportunities possible for healthy development. The book is based in the belief that change is possible, whether it is facilitated at the level of society, of community, within the family or by individuals themselves. Resilience is a current theme. One very influential theory of child development is Bronfenbrenner's (1979) ecological model of human development. It is particularly influential in the thinking that underpins *From Birth to Sixteen* since it takes account of development in a range of different contexts and does not only focus on individual characteristics of the child or young person. Ecology here refers to the environmental settings which the child or young person is experiencing or is linked to, directly and indirectly. Bronfenbrenner proposed that individuals develop in four nested systems:

- *Microsystem* – this inner level refers to the experiences of the individual in a particular setting. For the young child, this is usually the home environment; for the older child or young person, this may be the school environment, with teachers and peers.
- *Mesosystem* – this next level refers to links and interactions among settings that the individual directly participates in. For example, the quality of the child's home environment might affect his or her academic performance in school or the nature of peer relationships.
- *Exosystem* – this level refers to links with settings that the individual does not participate in directly but which have an influence on that person's life. For example, the parent's work environment may affect their physical health or their emotional well-being and so influence the quality of the care that they provide for their child.
- *Macrosystem* – this level refers to the general pattern of ideology and organization of social institutions in the wider society in which the individual exists. So, for example, the effects of parental stress at work, or the impact of unemployment, or the outbreak of war or social unrest, will have an impact on the growing child.

Bronfenbrenner argued that changes in one level of the system could have a huge impact on other levels. For example, recession in the wider society (the *macrosystem*) can affect the parent's work experience (the *exosystem*) and so impact on the quality of the family's life (the *mesosystem*) and in turn affect the health and emotional well-being of the child. From this perspective, in order to understand the processes of child development fully, we must take account of the complex interactions among the different levels of the system. This is particularly important when we try to make changes in the child's life or to undo damage that has occurred in the past. In fact, an essential part of development is the ability to cope with the inevitable changes that will happen in the course of life.

From Birth to Sixteen has many examples of interventions designed to improve the lives of children and young people. For example, European initiatives, such as EU Kids Online, alert us to the danger that young people face on the internet and recommend action that might be taken to prevent it happening and to buffer the negative effects. Nationwide interventions such as the Social and Emotional Aspects of Learning (SEAL) curriculum aim to teach children the skills of emotional literacy. Campaigns like the Teenage Pregnancy Independent Advisory Group (TPIAG) chart some success in reducing the numbers of unplanned births to very young mothers. Smaller-scale interventions pioneer new methods. For example, *Linking Lies* (Jennifer & Williams, 2011) provides guidance on how to use restorative methods for addressing sexual bullying and gender conflict among young people.

Research gives key signposts for the practitioner. The English and Romanian Adoptees (ERA) project provides longitudinal data about the adoption into UK families of children who had been severely neglected in Romanian orphanages. Initiatives, such as the Nurture Group Network, evaluate intervention to help insecurely attached children reintegrate with their families and their peers at school. Sure Start outcomes indicate the crucial importance of high-quality provision for pre-school children. Research plays a key part in guiding professional practice, and, wherever possible, the interventions described in this book have been systematically evaluated.

Chapter 2 focuses on the evolving sense of self and others from the moment of birth right through to identity formation in adolescence, and charts the crucial role that adults play in their everyday interactions, playful encounters and chats in facilitating healthy growth. Methods for promoting emotional literacy at school are also discussed, as well as specialist provision for children with emotional and behavioural difficulties.

Chapter 3 examines attachments within the family and charts the development of relationships with different family members and caregivers. It also examines the emotional impact on the child and young person resulting from the loss of a significant adult. The effects of severe early neglect are illustrated by the ERA study of Romanian adoptees and the case study of a looked-after child.

Chapter 4 examines children's experiences of day care and nursery school, and explores the evidence about the stages at which young children can be deemed to be ready to be cared for outside the home. This chapter also emphasizes the critical importance of peer relationships at pre-school and school. The issue of in-groups and out-groups is discussed in the context of the processes of change, over time and in different socio-historic contexts, of children's ethnic and national identities. The issue of bullying and social exclusion is also considered. Moving on to adolescence, the chapter explores the changing nature of peer relationships, including sexual/romantic relationships. This chapter ends by looking at violent, antisocial behaviour in school and in the community as well as the counterbalancing phenomenon of prosocial activity on the part of young people.

Chapter 5 begins with an overview of major theories of language development and discusses some of the ongoing controversies in this field. Cross-cultural studies provide challenging evidence about the processes of language development in the child. The chapter returns to the influence of close relationships with adults in guiding the development of language and communication skills throughout childhood and adolescence. It documents the importance of shared narratives in fostering the mind-mindedness that underpins the development of language. The chapter also explores some of the difficulties faced by children who enter school without pre-reading and pre-writing skills and identifies some of the interventions that teachers can implement.

Chapter 6 looks at the impact of traditional and new media – including television, advertising, video games, internet, e-mail, blogs and chat rooms – on the lives of children and young people. It explores the benefits as well as major risks, and includes current research and policy on safer use of the internet.

Chapter 7 explores the health risks for children and young people that arise from excessive use of alcohol, drugs and other substances, as well as some effective interventions to counteract this disturbing trend. The chapter continues by examining another major health risk in today's society – the growing incidence of obesity – and its impact on the health and emotional well-being of children and young people. It ends with an overview of common eating disorders and describes therapeutic interventions to help young people and their families to overcome these disorders as well as educational programmes that schools can implement to heighten awareness of the problem and promote healthy eating patterns.

The focus of Chapter 8 is on safe and risky sexual behaviour. This chapter includes typical sexual behaviour as well as aspects of precocious and problematic sexual behaviour. It examines common health risks arising from unprotected sex, including sexually transmitted infections and unplanned pregnancy. Interventions to promote sexual health are included.

Finally, Chapter 9 explores methods for addressing emotional and behavioural difficulties in childhood and adolescence and looks at how to promote emotional health and well-being.

Further reading

There are useful government reports on health in childhood and adolescence, these include: Department of Health/Department of Education (2009) *Healthy Lives, Brighter Futures: The Strategy for Young People's Health*, London: HMSO.

An excellent resource for clinical practice, that covers common paediatric disorders from birth to adolescence, is: Rudolf, M., Lee, T. & Levene, M. (2011) *Paediatrics and Child Health*, 3rd edition, Chichester: Wiley/Blackwell.

Another useful health resource, specifically designed for nursing, is: Davies, R. & Davies, A. (eds) (2011) *Children and Young People's Nursing: Principles for Practice*, London: Hodder Arnold.

For an up-to-date account of adolescent development, see: Coleman, J. (2011) *The Nature of Adolescence*, 4th edition, Hove: Psychology Press.

For a detailed and knowledgeable account of interventions to address social disadvantage, read: Belsky, J., Barnes, J. & Melhuish, E. (2007) *The National Evaluation of Sure Start: Does Area-based Early Intervention Work?* Bristol: The Policy Press.

The league tables of inequality are reported in detail in: UNICEF (2010) *The Children Left Behind: A League Table of Inequality in Child Well-being in the World's Richest Countries*, Innocenti Report Card 9, Florence: UNICEF Innocenti Research Centre.

Redsell, S. & Hastings, A. (eds) (2010) *Listening to Children and Young People in Healthcare Consultations*, Abingdon: Radcliffe, has contributions from a range of healthcare professionals, including paediatricians, midwives, health visitors, general practitioners, nurses and psychologists, and offers perspectives on engagement and communication on the part of healthcare professionals with children and young people within health and social care contexts.

Chapter 2

The evolving sense of self and others

Map of the chapter

In the early part of a child's life there is very little differentiation between self and other. This chapter explores the processes through which the child's and adolescent's sense of self evolves. The capacity for experiencing empathy for others' feelings plays a particularly important role in this process. The chapter charts key changes in the child's sense of self as a separate entity from that of others, and discusses the nature of self-concept and self-esteem at different stages in childhood and adolescence. Self-esteem is widely associated with academic achievement, social competence and emotional well-being. As a result, many interventions have been created to enhance the self-esteem of children and young people. Primary prevention programmes focus on the whole population while treatment programmes focus on children and young people with particular needs. Illustrations of each are described in this chapter. The large literature in this field provides evidence to support the use of humanistic, child-centred approaches for the care and education of children and young people, with a particular focus on the role of emotions and relationships in the development of the self.

Self-concept and emotions

The child's sense of self is closely related to the ways in which he or she expresses and interprets emotions. From the moment of birth babies signal their emotional state whether they are content (slight smiles) or distressed (pursed lips, mouth down). Parents/carers report that they can distinguish a range of basic emotions in their baby during the first few months of life, including happiness, interest, surprise, sadness, fear, anger and pain. Babies also seem to show the capacity to recognize and interpret the emotions of others from a very early age. They can mimic the facial gestures of another person, for example sticking out the tongue or opening the mouth. By 10 weeks, they can imitate the basic features of the mother's emotional expressions of anger and happiness (Haviland & Lelwica, 1987).

Traditional views of emotions considered them as subjective states that existed quite separately from thinking, language and behaviour, but more recent theory and research suggests that emotions have many aspects, each part of a dynamic system that is connected to other psychological processes, and intricately involved with the quality of relationships with caring adults. Here is how Fernyhough (2008: 46) describes the emotions expressed by Athena in the first few weeks of her life:

> She gives as well as receiving. She has expectations of how I will behave, and she reacts if I don't fulfil them. She can recognize a few different emotional expressions, and reproduce the most basic ones for herself. If I were to change my expression suddenly from happy to angry, for example, she would show surprise. If I suddenly made my face freeze up altogether, she would stop smiling, look away and then try to re-engage my attention.

The responsiveness of the adult is crucial. Meins *et al.* (2002) suggest that parents' **mind-mindedness** is crucial from the earliest years. Mind-mindedness refers to the way that a parent treats their infant as an individual with a mind, rather than as a creature with needs to be met. The emphasis here is on responding to the child's inferred state of mind rather than only on their behaviour.

As the example of Athena shows, babies are also attuning themselves to the adults. Psychologists (e.g., Mumme & Fernald, 2003) call this *social referencing*, a process through which the infant will look carefully at the mother/caregiver as if to gauge their emotional expression before responding to a situation or object. The process continues. Moses *et al.* (2001) found that infants of 12–18 months, when given a strange toy, would often look at the adult as if checking how to react. Then they would use the adult's words, for example, 'Wow!' or 'Nice!' for positive feelings, and 'Yuk!' or 'Yeech!' for negative feelings.

There are wide variations in the extent to which parents/carers comment appropriately on their babies' internal states, but there is evidence that sensitive attunement on the part of the adult to the babies' emotional state has long-term effects on the child's development of a sense of self. Meins *et al.* (2002) reported a link between maternal mind-mindedness when their children were five months and superior performance by the child at age 4 years on **theory of mind** tasks (that is, tasks that assess the child's capacity to attribute mental states, such as beliefs, desires and intentions, to themselves and others) (see Box 2.2). The mothers who commented appropriately on their infants' state of mind during free play indicated these mothers' ability to 'read' their babies' emotional states accurately. Examples of this included commenting that the child was content while playing quietly with a toy or that the baby was thinking while he/she looked pensive. By contrast, some mothers appeared to misread their babies' internal states. For example, they said that their baby was bored when the baby was actually playing quietly but happily.

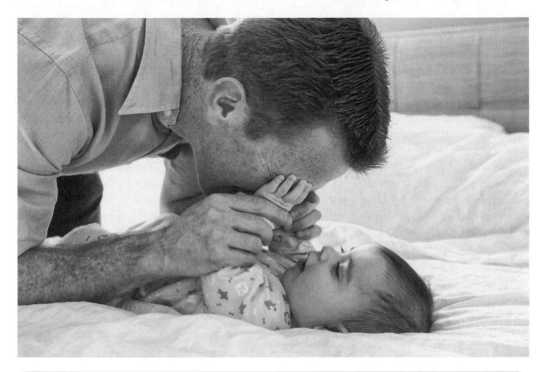

Marcy Maloy/Getty images

Awareness of self and others

Self-concept can be usefully divided into three interrelated aspects: **self-image, self-esteem** and **ideal self. Self-image** usually refers to the descriptive way in which a person portrays or represents him/herself, often in terms of their social identity (e.g., 'I am a mother' or 'I am Welsh'), their personality (e.g., 'I am a calm person') or their physical appearance (e.g., 'I am a fat person'). But there is another important dimension to the self – **self-esteem** – which refers to the extent to which a person values the self, with all its attributes and characteristics. So 'I am Welsh' could be a statement laden with pride in one's ethnicity, while 'I am a fat person' could represent a negative view of oneself as too big in comparison with others. The terms self-concept and self-esteem are often used interchangeably in the literature since the subjective meanings of self-description and self-evaluation overlap. The **ideal self** refers to the person whom we aspire to be. Some people are content with the person they are; others are perpetually striving to be someone completely different. The presence of an ideal self can be very motivating in terms of self-development or career aspiration but, if the discrepancy between self-image and ideal self is too great, then self-esteem is likely to be lower. In each aspect, the social context is very relevant as the person internalizes the experiences and values of family, community and society, and reflects on the self in relation to significant others in their world.

In general, children and adolescents are motivated to maintain self-esteem as a protection against threats to the self, such as anxiety. Self-esteem is also closely related to the person's sense of belongingness as it provides feedback on how that person is valued and accepted by the people that matter most. When adults are nurturing and approving of the child in their care, they are much more likely to build up the child's self-esteem than are adults who are disapproving, unresponsive and uninterested. By adolescence, the peer group becomes increasingly important to the young person. Approval and acceptance by peers becomes the most important influence on self-esteem.

Mead (1934) developed his influential theory of **symbolic interactionism** on the basis that there is a distinction between the 'I' (self as knower) and the 'me' (self as known). Mead proposed a reflexive process through which we stand back from the self in order to interact with it and experience it. The symbolic interactionist stance proposes that the self-concept evolves when the child takes the perspective of significant others in his/her life and so comes to see the self as an object – that is, sees him/herself through the eyes of others. It is through this process of 'objectifying' the self that the self-concept develops. If a child has positive self-esteem, this is often taken to be an essential ingredient for emotional health and well-being. Self-esteem depends very much on the relationships that the child experiences with significant others in his/her social world. From the symbolic interactionist perspective, developing children are, from the beginning, active agents in the long process of learning about the social and emotional world that they inhabit. As indicated earlier, it is a two-way process in which adults' and children's attunement to one another is critical. Significant adults in the child's world play a crucial role in providing the kind of nurturing, supportive environment in which children can grow socially and emotionally.

More recently, Hoffman (2000: 64) proposes that there are four broad stages in the development of the child's concept of self and other:

- unclear or confused differentiation between self and other;
- awareness of self and others as separate physical entities;
- awareness of self and others as having independent internal states;
- awareness of self and others as having their own histories, identities and lives beyond the immediate situation.

Hoffman's model proposes that these social-cognitive stages interact with the child's emerging sense of **empathy**. He defines empathy as the emotion that a person feels as appropriate for another's situation, not one's own. The capacity for experiencing feelings of empathic awareness of another person's situation develops over time, but it is present in a very basic form from the early days of a child's life. These feelings are nurtured and fostered through the everyday interactions with significant others in the child's life.

The early years

The emergence of empathy

The newborn baby will cry when he/she hears another baby cry, as Darwin (1877) found in his detailed observations of his own son's behaviour from birth, and this crying is virtually indistinguishable from the child's own spontaneous cries of distress. Since the babies are responding to distress in another baby by feeling distressed themselves, this can be considered as a very rudimentary precursor of empathy (Hoffman, 2000). By six months, the nature of this response has changed. Darwin noted that his son at six months would first look sad and pucker up his lips before starting to cry when his nurse pretended to be upset. As we saw above, the infant is developing a sense of person permanence, that is, a sense that the other person is someone separate from himself, but the awareness is still tentative. At around 12 months, in addition to looking sad, puckering the lips and crying, babies will also engage in behaviour to alleviate *their own* distress. In other words, as Hoffman's (ibid.) theory proposes, they are demonstrating **egocentric empathic distress**, that is, showing signs of responding more actively to the distressing situation but still having difficulty in differentiating between the distress of another and their own:

> Empathic distress late in the first year is an egocentric motive but, unlike other egocentric motives, it is triggered by another's distress and this gives it prosocial properties. It is not a complete prosocial motive but is halfway there and could just as well be called a *precursor* of prosocial motivation.

> (ibid: 69–70)

Empathy is closely related to the development of the child's concept of self and, eventually, to the development of such abstract concepts as caring and justice.

Recognizing the self

At the beginning, the baby has no sense of difference between self and others and before this can happen the baby must develop the concept of **object permanence**, the understanding that something still exists, even when it is out of sight. Similarly, the understanding that other people have a separate and permanent existence has been defined as **person permanence**. In order to have the concept of person permanence, the baby must have some form of representation of the other as a person with an existence in time and space. One way of assessing person permanence is to observe babies' behaviour when a familiar person moves out of range, as in the game of 'Peekaboo'. From a very early age, infants will indicate that they have some sense of their separateness from the other by appearing to search for that person when they 'disappear'.

Fernyhough (2008: 123) describes how his daughter, Athena, at around four-and-a-half months, was fascinated by mirrors. Her parents would sit her on the bed and then stand to one side so that she could see them in the mirror but not herself. When they waved, she would wave back. Then she would turn to look at them in reality before looking again at their reflection, as if comparing the reality with the image.

Person permanence experiments indicate that the baby can recognize others and expect them to continue to exist. But what can we infer about the baby's emergent sense of self? Fernyhough (ibid.: 123–124) observed Athena at four-and-a-half months when she was held close to the mirror so that she could see her *own* reflection. First she stared at the image of herself, then glanced at the corners of the mirror as though checking out the nature of this new form of reality. Then she reached forward with excitement 'looking the reflected stranger up and down in what could almost be taken for suspicion'. Then she seemed to note the similarities between her own movements and those reflected in the mirror, suggesting that this image was in some way connected to her. But when Lizzie, her mother, put a smear of rouge on Athena's nose, the child did not pay any attention to the red blob on the nose of the reflected image. See how this understanding evolves in Case Study 2.1 and Box 2.1.

Athena recognizes herself in the mirror

It was not until she was around 14 months that she was able to name the baby in the mirror as 'Athena'. Then, when Lizzie put the blob of rouge on her nose, Athena showed her understanding that the reflection was herself:

> Her nose newly spotted, Athena looks back at her image, glances away, then does a double take, gazing back at herself with more purpose. She looks at her mother, touching her nose, then turns to the mirror again.
>
> 'Look!' she says, with genuine surprise.
>
> 'What is it?' Lizzie asks.
>
> Athena looks back with a big grin. The test has become a game. She bats at the spot in the mirror, then touches her own blotched features. She is doing something quite remarkable: seeing herself as others see her, and somehow identifying herself with the image.
>
> (ibid.: 124–125)

Discussion questions

At what point does an infant realize that the baby in the mirror is in fact the self? What is the evidence for this? Can we really know what is going on in a baby's mind?

Box 2.1

Assessing self-recognition in babies (Lewis & Brooks-Gunn, 1979)

This test of self-recognition was first developed by Lewis and Brooks-Gunn (ibid.) when they assessed 16 infants in six age groups: at 9, 12, 15, 18, 21 and 24 months. First, they arranged for the mothers to place their babies in front of a large mirror for about 90 seconds. At all ages, the babies in this study reached out to the mirror or pointed at it. Then each baby's nose was gently smeared with rouge and replaced in front of the mirror. The 9- and 12-month-old babies did not respond to this new condition; a minority of 15- and 18-month-old babies touched their own noses, as did most 21- and 24-month-old babies. The researchers concluded that by 18 months, most babies have a clear idea that the reflection in the mirror is a representation of themselves. By 15–18 months, most babies can use verbal labels (like 'baby') or their own name to distinguish between pictures of themselves and of other children of the same age. They smile more and look longer at pictures of themselves (ibid.). At around the same age, like Athena, they recognize themselves in a mirror, so indicating that they have a sense of self that can be represented outside their own body and can be seen by others.

Discussion questions

How far have the babies come in their awareness of the difference between self and other by the age of 2? Why is this self-awareness so important?

Developing a theory of mind

In order to appreciate that another person's knowledge, beliefs and desires are different from yours, you need to have the capacity for **mind-reading**, sometimes referred to as **theory of mind**, that is, the ability to attribute mental states to yourself as well as to others. Theory of mind can be considered as one of the most important attributes that humans possess. We engage in theory of mind routinely when we interact with others. We look at the other person's clothes and body language in order to decide what kind of individual they are and how we should approach them. If we get it wrong, we commit a social *faux pas* or worse. For example, Jane invited Susan round for dinner and served steak. She had forgotten that Susan was a committed vegetarian and was totally mortified by her social gaffe, since she had failed to show sensitivity to her friend's needs, likes and values.

Box 2.2

Assessing a child's theory of mind (Harris, 1989)

Harris demonstrated that pre-school children are able to mind-read other people's emotions, desires and beliefs, as he demonstrated by means of theory of mind tasks. He and his co-researchers asked children to listen to stories about imaginary characters, Ellie the elephant, who had very particular likes and dislikes, and Mickey the monkey, who was very mischievous. Some children were told that Ellie the elephant only liked to drink milk and others were told that she only liked to drink Coke. Then they were told that Mickey the monkey, for a joke, emptied the Coke can and filled it up with milk. The children were then asked how Ellie the elephant would feel when she tasted her drink. Four-year-olds were able to answer correctly that (if she likes milk) she will be pleased, or that (if she likes Coke) she will be sad, and explain why in terms of Ellie's preferences, not their own.

Harris argues that once children are aware of their own emotional state, they can use their imagination to project emotional states onto other people or imaginary characters and, through this process, gradually come to understand that other people's imagined worlds may differ from their own.

Discussion questions

Why would 2-year-olds find this task hard? Think of other ways in which you might assess a child's capacity to mind-read.

Harris (ibid.) proposed that the child's awareness of their own mental state enables them to project mental states onto the other person. They do this, according to Harris's theory, by a process of imagining themselves in the other person's position. We see the process in motion when we read stories with young children by entering into the mental models that seem to underpin the child's responses to the narrative. These responses indicate the child's creation of an imaginary world. Harris (2000) argues that the ability to construct models of events that are not immediately visible in our 'real' world evolved from humans' need to process language in all its forms. Making sense of an imaginary story-world helps the child to understand past and future, and to imagine things that might be possible. Fernyhough (2008: 171) calls it 'mental time travel' which the child can operate in forward and reverse gear. As Harris (1989) argues, there are three important preconditions that enable the child to understand another person's world:

Box 2.3

Preconditions for understanding the world of another person (derived from Harris, 1989)

Self-awareness: by 18–20 months most children are aware of themselves, and by two years they have the words to express their emotional states.

Capacity for pretence: by 2–3 years, children spend a great deal of time engaged in pretend play. They will act out role-plays with dolls and stuffed toys. These characters will have desires and emotions of their own (see Case Study 2.2).

Distinguishing reality from pretence: out of the capacity for pretence develops the ability to distinguish clearly between what is real and what is imaginary. By 3–4 years, this understanding is usually stable.

CASE STUDY 2.2

Yasmin's understanding of emotions

Yasmin, aged 3 years, has set out a teaset in front of her family of toy rabbits. As she plays, she enacts different scenes. Each character has a different voice and they each express different emotions. In one scene, Little Rabbit has spilled his tea on the tablecloth. Mrs Rabbit tells him off. Yasmin comments, as narrator, that 'Little Rabbit spilled his tea. Mummy Rabbit was very cross. He's sad now.' She makes Little Rabbit cry noisily.

Discussion questions

Does Yasmin show that she understands what sadness is? How does she link her own experience of being sad with the pretend play situation? How well is she interpreting Little Rabbit's emotional state?

By engaging in such commonplace activities as chatting about the events of the day, children are being enabled to think about the present in relation to past and future. There is evidence that adults can significantly influence the child's development of a theory of mind in enjoyable everyday conversations and activities. Fernyhough (2008: 170) gives detailed examples of these dialogues with his very young daughter beginning with such simple structures as: 'There was once a little girl called Athena who lived with her Mummy and Daddy in a house with a yellow door . . .'. As he points out, this method worked like magic for Athena since it gave her the opportunity to recount perspectives of her own world as seen through her eyes. The events of her day were told in a form of narrative in which, through the child/parent dialogue, the time and scene were set ('It was this morning'; 'We were at the shops') and the various characters were given emotions and motives.

Nelson and Fivush (2000) demonstrate that when parents/carers encourage toddlers from two years on to tell and retell narratives about past events in their lives, the children gradually become more and more sophisticated in their ability to recall details of the events and the emotions experienced by the people involved. Furthermore, the more that parents/carers support these dialogues, the more accomplished these children become when tested some years later. During the pre-school years, toddlers gradually come to understand and express the causes of emotions ('Ezra crying because his mummy gone away'), to link actions with emotional outcomes ('Why are you mad at me? What did I do?') and to interpret the facial expressions of other people ('Ellie's got a happy face 'cos she saw her granny').

Verbal deception

One interesting aspect of this process is the evolving capacity that children have to deceive others. In order to deceive another person successfully, you need to have a theory of the other person's mind, so lie-tellers need to regulate their expressive behaviours in order to avoid inconsistencies between their behaviour and the lie. There are two aspects: *verbal expressive behaviour* (the content of the statements that children make during deception) and *non-verbal expressive behaviour* (their facial expression and body language). When children lie, they must ensure that the content of the verbal statement they make does not contradict the lie. Talwar and Lee (2002) call this *semantic leakage control*. Children who lie must also simulate non-verbal behaviours that are consistent with the untruthful statements and suppress spontaneous non-verbal responses that might show that they are lying. This is categorized as *non-verbal leakage control*. Children tell lies, just as adults do, for a number of reasons – to spare people's feelings, to avoid disapproval or punishment, to give a good impression and for gain (see Box 2.4).

Box 2.4

Testing children's ability to deceive (Talwar & Lee, 2002)

Talwar and Lee (ibid.) designed an experiment to test young children's ability to use verbal and non-verbal leakage control in order to deceive adults. The researchers created what they called a *temptation resistance* procedure. Children aged from 3 to 7 years played a guessing game in which they had to guess the names of hidden toys. Finally, they were told not to peek at a music-playing toy located behind them while the experimenter was out of the room. But most children could not resist the temptation and peeked. When the experimenter returned, the children were asked if they had peeked. The researchers predicted that children would lie in the temptation resistance situation and that the number of lie-tellers would increase with age. They also predicted that the lie-tellers' ability to mask their non-verbal expressive behaviour would also increase with age. They found that, in the temptation resistance situation, most children peeked when they had been asked not to. They could not resist the temptation to look at the hidden toy while the experimenter was out of the room. The majority lied when asked by the experimenter if they had peeked, with the exception of the 3-year-olds, a third

---

of whom confessed that they had peeked. The findings indicate that lying behaviour increases rapidly during the pre-school years. Most adults, when asked to decide whether the children were lying or not, could not discriminate the lie-tellers from non-liars on the basis of their non-verbal expressive behaviour. At the same time, many of the children were unskilled at semantic leakage control so that adults could easily identify the lie-tellers on the basis of their verbal statements made in the same context as the lie. Talwar and Lee (ibid.) conclude that children as young as 3 years can lie to conceal a transgression. It can be hard for adults to tell if they are lying from their non-verbal expressive behaviour, but when the children are questioned they are not so good at managing their semantic leakage. Therefore adults can more easily work out that they are lying.

Discussion questions

Why were the younger children less expert at responding verbally than non-verbally when trying to hide their deception? What does this tell us about their capacity to read the minds of others?

The primary school years

Developing empathic awareness

At the beginning of this period, children typically demonstrate a deeper understanding of the relationship between their own feelings and those of others. By 6 or 7 years of age, they are becoming aware of the value of friendship and the range of feelings involved in close relationships. They also demonstrate their knowledge that they can comfort a person in distress. Many children seem to have more awareness and self-reflectiveness about the meaning of their own feelings when in the presence of another person who is suffering or when they experience a character's emotions in literature or in the media.

By 8 or 9 years of age, children can describe complex, opposing feelings, for example when a person is happy to see someone in hospital but at the same time sad because that person is ill. They can speculate about how another person might feel; for example, a child might be feeling unappreciated because they have low self-esteem even though they played well in a team. Hoffman (2000: 76) describes a study in which children were asked to say how angry they would be at someone who, for example, stole their cat. They were then given extenuating circumstances about the perpetrator's life (for example, that his own cat had run away and his parents would not buy him a new one). Those who were 8 years and older were much more likely to state that they would be less angry than same-age children who were given a similar amount of background information about the perpetrator but without the extenuating circumstances. Younger children were unaffected by the knowledge of the perpetrator's life difficulties and made no concessions.

Regulating emotions

Throughout the primary school years, children come to understand about the management of emotions in more complex ways than they did in the pre-school years. For example, 6-year-olds understand that a child can look happy, even though she does not feel happy, because she does not want others to know about her inner state. Most emotional regulation is learned informally through myriad interactions with family members, siblings and peers. The process of emotional regulation evolves as a way of managing relationships and dealing with the ups and downs of everyday life. Primary school children learn that what is appropriate for a toddler may not be acceptable once you go to school. Throwing a tantrum when you do not get what you want is likely to be met with derision by school friends so most children quickly learn 'appropriate' ways of expressing what they feel.

There may well be a cost attached to emotional regulation. Escobar *et al.* (2011) found that children with low self-esteem or those who were rejected by their peers were more likely to be perceived as 'demanding' or 'needy' if they sought social support when they were bullied or socially excluded. Similarly, Mahady Wilton *et al.* (2000) found that if bullied children expressed their distress too openly, they were unlikely to get support; in fact, the bullying might increase. Learning to regulate emotions is an essential developmental task if children are to cope with the complex array of situations, some very stressful, that they will inevitably encounter in their lives. In the pre-school years parents/caregivers are there to help them manage their feelings. But, as they grow older, they are increasingly reliant on relationships with peers and on the quality of the school's support systems for helping them to develop coping strategies for managing emotions. The capacity for self-regulation can have far-reaching effects in adolescence and beyond.

Self-concept and self-esteem

Self-esteem, as the child's subjective evaluation of his/her worth as a person, can be both specific to one domain (e.g., 'I believe that I am good at maths') and can be global (e.g., 'I feel proud that I am an honest person'). Self-esteem in many studies has been linked with happiness and emotional well-being. Some self-esteem researchers have proposed a global model as an overall positive or negative view of the self. Others prefer to explain self-esteem in terms of a multidimensional model, in which self-concept comes to represent perceptions of competence in, for example, social, behavioural and academic spheres. For a useful discussion of these debates, see Harter (1985), Marsh and Craven (2006) and Swann *et al.* (2007).

By the time they enter primary school, most children can express some form of specific, though not always accurate, self-evaluation. But, as they enter a wider range of domains in their social and academic world, they become more able to express descriptions and judgements about such dimensions as the active self and the social self (Box 2.5). Harter (1999) proposed that two factors play a significant role in the development of self-esteem: *perceived competence* in areas of importance and the *experience of social support*. Good academic performance is more likely to win the approval of parents and teachers; good physical appearance, prowess at sports and popularity with peers are more likely to result in the approval of other children. Harter (ibid.) found a change in children's self-concept during the primary school years as the sometimes unrealistic self-perceptions of early childhood give way to more accurate perceptions of abilities and competences, as internalized by information from many sources.

As children develop, they become more able to be self-critical in judging their own efforts and abilities. These appraisals of self are, inevitably, linked to self-esteem. In order to feel positively about themselves, children need to feel that they are competent in the areas that are important to them, as well as to significant others in their lives, whether adults or peers. For example, a child might perceive that he is very competent at sports and feel very happy when involved in team activities with his classmates. The fact that he is not outstanding academically would not necessarily detract from his high self-esteem since the significant people in his life regularly affirm his success in the areas that really matter to him. So feeling a lack of competence in one domain does not automatically lead to lowered self-esteem, provided that meaningful protective factors are in place. Similarly, a child might say, realistically, 'I am useless at netball!' but this lack of competence in one specific domain need not impinge on the child's overall self-esteem since playing netball, in this case, was not a central part of the child's life. Tatlow-Golden and Guerin (2010) use a multidimensional model to elicit children's own views of the active and social self, as discussed in Box 2.5.

Box 2.5

Exploring children's self-concept (adapted from Tatlow-Golden & Guerin, 2010)

In this study, the researchers investigated the use of a qualitative method for giving insight into children's self-concept by inviting 125 Irish children aged 10–13 years of age (73 boys and 52 girls) to draw and write about their favourite people and things to do. The researchers employed a multidimensional model of the self in which self-evaluation is measured in specific domains rather than as a global concept. Qualitative measures have great potential in accessing the richness of children's concept of self. In this study, the researchers focused on children's *active* (favourite activity) and *social* (favourite person) self-concept. The children were invited to 'draw a picture of yourself doing your favourite thing. It can be something you do at home, at school or anything else . . . You decide!' At the bottom of the page, the children were invited to include written comments.

Active self
With regard to the active self, there were two main categories: physical activities and non-physical activities.

Physical activities: two-thirds of participants represented themselves doing something physically active, including football, ice skating, gymnastics, skipping. Significantly fewer girls drew team sports (e.g., football, hockey) as their favourite activity (32.7%) than boys (54.8%). By contrast, more girls (23.1%) chose non-sport activities (e.g., skateboarding, ice-skating) than boys (9.6%). But overall, when all physical categories were combined, boys and girls did not differ.

Non-physical activities: just over half of the children drew and wrote about other active-self factors such as playing a musical instrument, baking, playing computer games.

The children's written comments concerned fitness and friendship, enjoyment, fun, relaxation and play. Competitiveness did not feature at all.

Social self

Family and friends featured frequently, including a wide range of immediate and extended family members, godparents and best friends. In their comments, children elaborated on the meaning that these relationships had for them in terms of emotional and social support. Seven per cent of the sample chose pets as their favourite 'people'. For example, one 12-year-old boy drew pictures of his cousin and his hamster, describing them as his two best friends and as 'the people I like the most'; one 11-year-old girl identified her cat as her 'favourite person' because of its ability to 'understand what I say'. Ten per cent of boys (but no girls) chose celebrities or fictional heroes as their favourite people.

The researchers conclude that traditional adult-constructed self-esteem scales may underestimate the scope and richness of children's self-concept in both the physical and social domains. Typical self-esteem scales question children about *team* sports yet the present study revealed the significance of *non-team* sport activity as well. Among other things, this means that girls' physical self-esteem may be underestimated in many studies using standard self-esteem scales. In terms of social self, the present study indicated a wide definition of family and friends to include people beyond the immediate nuclear family, as well as the emotionally important value of pets.

Child-centred methods like draw-and-write give deep insights into the child's concept of self. This knowledge is needed if adults are to develop effective interventions to promote self-esteem. The findings indicate the value of examining children's distinctive interests (both in the active and the social self) rather than focusing only on global measures.

Discussion questions

Why is it so important to consult with children in order to understand the developing self? Can you think of other qualitative methods that could be used?

Adolescence

A time of transition

The transition from childhood to adolescence brings dramatic changes in self-concept. Research studies document a decrease in self-esteem at this point and suggest a number of reasons for the change. For one thing, boys and girls are socially, cognitively and emotionally affected by transition from primary to secondary school (see Chapter 4). At the same time, they are experiencing the physical and emotional changes that take place during puberty. Whereas before puberty most children feel comfortable with their bodies, in early adolescence young people become much more conscious of their body image, its shape, size and appearance, and frequently experience dissatisfaction with it (see Chapter 7). At this stage, there is often a discrepancy between the ideal self (e.g., as portrayed by the media) and the young person's self-concept. In addition, since they spend more time with their peers, they are likely to become preoccupied with friendships and with romantic and sexual relationships. As a result, they become increasingly concerned about acceptance within the peer group and run the risk of being vulnerable to feelings of isolation or rejection when relationships do not work out well. Gender differences are evident at this stage, with girls being more vulnerable to lower self-esteem than boys (Harter, 1999).

Identity formation

A key psychosocial theory of the self is that of Erikson (1968) who proposed that at each stage of development the person has a particular task to achieve and an identity crisis to overcome. Erikson argued that the search for identity is especially acute during adolescence because of rapid biological and social changes at this time. With particular reference to adolescence, some form of crisis resolution is essential if the young person is to form an identity and to defeat **identity diffusion**. Erikson viewed four aspects of identity diffusion as consisting of:

1 the challenge of intimacy (including a longing for close relationships as well as a fear of commitment);
2 the diffusion of time perspective (including difficulties in planning for the future);
3 the diffusion of industry (including the challenge of harnessing personal resources to prepare for adult life); and
4 the concept of negative identity (choosing an identity that challenges the beliefs of parents or other important adults).

Strongly influenced by Erikson's (ibid.) theory, Marcia (1993) identified four critical states (rather than stages) in the process of identity formation during adolescence:

- **Identity diffusion**: the young person is in crisis and finds it difficult to achieve a clear sense of self-concept;
- **Identity foreclosure**: the young person avoids the uncertainty and anxiety of crisis by committing themselves to safe, conventional goals without exploring the many options open to them;
- **Identity moratorium**: the young person postpones making decisions about their identity and experiments with a range of roles. They might, for example, experiment with different sexual and romantic partners. They might rebel against adult values by identifying with rebellious groups. They might dress in provocative, challenging ways;
- **Identity achievement**: the young person emerges from the struggle to form an identity with clear commitments, goals, values and aspirations.

These identity states can be viewed in a developmental sequence but they do not necessarily occur in stages. However, Marcia (ibid.) proposed that some form of moratorium was necessary for identity achievement. For further discussion, see also Kroger (2004).

The capacity for empathy

By early adolescence, young people are developing more sophisticated self-awareness than they had in primary school, for example, compassion for another's distress combined with awareness of the need to proceed with sensitivity when offering support. Research into peer support indicates children's capacity to be sensitive to a much wider range of emotions when helping vulnerable people, such as pupils who are being socially excluded by their classmates. Adolescents demonstrate that they are able to experience feelings of compassion alongside an awareness that their empathy for the person in distress can be shown in a number of ways depending on the needs of the other and the context of where they are. Cowie and Olafsson (2000) interviewed pupils in a secondary school set in a disadvantaged inner-city catchment area with very high levels of aggression and violence. A selected group of volunteers aged 13–15 years had been trained in peer support skills by an experienced counsellor. Case Study 2.3 gives extracts from the interviews that demonstrate their sensitivity and skill in offering help to vulnerable peers:

CASE STUDY 2.3

Supporting peers in distress (from Cowie & Olafsson, 2000: 87)

'They tell us their problem and we summarize what they say. And eye contact, body contact, all counts. This makes them feel that we are actually listening and that we're interested . . . and we're there to help them out' (Delroy, a peer supporter).

'I passed by and saw him very upset, and I was concerned, so I went over there to talk to him. So, from then, I got him referred (to the peer support service) and I took him through the procedure of confidentiality, and told him how to sort out his problem and what he can do . . . (now) he says, "Hello" to me, I say, "Hello" to him . . . and he's got plenty of friends' (Hussein, a peer supporter).

Discussion questions

How do the peer supporters express their empathy for peers in distress? How might their actions contribute to their own sense of self-esteem?

Narcissism: false self-esteem

By contrast with the prosocial peer supporters whose actions not only help others but, in the process, foster high self-esteem, there are narcissistic young people who seem on the surface to be self-confident with high levels of self-esteem but who are often considered by peers to be egotistical and conceited individuals with a grandiose conception of themselves. This has been defined as **narcissism** or **false self-esteem**. Narcissism and positive self-esteem could at first sight seem to be very similar. But narcissism, unlike true self-esteem, is characterized by what Baumeister *et al.* (1996) call *defensive egotism* – a tendency to hold favourable self-appraisals that may be not grounded in reality or may be exaggerated, combined with difficulty in accepting any criticism. Threats to such self-appraisals are met with aggression. Narcissistic individuals demonstrate self-preoccupation, a need to seek out attention, excessive admiration of the self and a heightened concern to win approval from important others. Narcissism can be observed in the behaviour of some very aggressive people whose belief systems emphasize their superiority over others (Baumeister, 2001; Daly, 2006). It is at the point at which such a person's self-appraisal is perceived to be under threat that they become aggressive. Daly (ibid.), in his study of 1,628 adolescents in six Australian schools, tested the hypothesis that high self-esteem, in conjunction with high levels of narcissism, would predict greater levels of bullying. The adolescents in this survey who scored highly on measures of self-esteem and narcissism also scored highly on aggression. His findings challenged the commonly held view that bullies use aggression to bolster their low self-esteem, and he concluded that a productive way forward for these aggressive young people would be to devise methods for enhancing their under-developed feelings of empathy for others.

Strategies for supporting self-esteem

The emotions continue to play a key role in the ways in which adults and young people work, interact and learn together (Cefai & Cooper, 2009; Hoffman, 2000) and to have a strong influence on the quality of interpersonal relationships in the peer group. Children and young people need to be equipped with emotional competence if they are to function effectively in their society. This means that adolescents, like younger children, must continue to understand and regulate their own emotions as well as develop empathy for the emotions of others. This process has been defined as the development of **emotional intelligence** (Goleman, 1995; Salovey & Mayer, 1990) or **emotional literacy** (Weare, 2004). Earlier experiences in the management of emotions are also relevant at this stage, as shown in Box 2.6.

Box 2.6

The long-term effects of self-control (Moffitt *et al.*, 2011)

Moffitt and her team investigated the self-control of 1,000 New Zealand children at the ages of 3, 5, 7, 9 and 11 years and then interviewed them when they reached the age of 32 years. The participants with low self-control as children were more likely as adults to be in a single-parent situation, to have money and health problems, and more likely to have been convicted of a criminal offence, even after adjusting for the effects of academic achievement and social class. The top fifth of the sample in terms of childhood self-control had rates of serious adult health problems of 11% as compared with 27% for

---

the bottom fifth of the sample. The crime rates in adulthood were 13% for those with high childhood self-control and 43% for those with low childhood self-control. There were also adolescent 'snares' which could trap individuals in harmful lifestyles. Children with low self-control in childhood were more likely to smoke in adolescence, to leave school with no qualifications and to become pregnant during adolescence. In turn, the 'snares' in adolescence predicted the chances of being in poor health and having money problems in adulthood.

The researchers conclude that intervention programmes should be designed to prevent situations that are likely to lead to lowered self-esteem in the primary school. Instead, school should boost self-esteem by creating caring communities that promote prosocial values and provide opportunities to practice self-management. This becomes even more important during adolescence when young people are more likely to be experimenting with different roles and engaging in risky behaviour. Intervention at this stage can help to prevent or at least ameliorate potentially life-changing outcomes. (See also Chapter 7 on alcohol and substance abuse, and Chapter 8 on teenage pregnancy.)

Discussion questions

Are there any other explanations for these findings, for example, the quality of family life, or stresses in the child's community? Would it be more helpful to intervene at an earlier age? Why might some adolescents have less self-control than others?

Harter (1999) has identified strategies for supporting the self-esteem of children and young people:

- *Reduce discrepancies* between aspirations (ideal self) and perceived competence (self-concept). This can be done by improving the young person's skills in areas where they feel that they are inadequate.
- *Highlight areas of competence* where the young person is skilled and help the young person to discount those areas where they perceive themselves to be less successful.
- *Develop emotional literacy* through programmes that provide opportunities for young people to develop self-awareness, self-confidence, insight into emotions, self-regulation and empathy for others.
- *Target low self-esteem* in vulnerable young people, help them to reframe their negative attributions of self and practise behavioural techniques for building self-confidence.

The next section gives examples of general emotional literacy programmes that aim to increase self-esteem, and prosocial behaviour, to reduce aggression and to enhance young people's capacity to relate well to one another.

The promotion of emotional health and well-being

Building on the research findings that link self-esteem to academic performance, social competence and emotional well-being, there exist a great variety of interventions designed to change self-esteem in children and young people. These interventions can be broadly divided into two main categories: i) emotional literacy programmes (sometimes referred to as primary prevention programmes) that enhance self-esteem and promote emotional health and well-being in all children and young people; and ii) programmes that target children and young people with specific social, behavioural and emotional needs.

In schools, there are a number of emotional literacy initiatives to promote emotional health and well-being among all pupils (Weare, 2004). These approaches are grounded in the belief that they develop skills that are fundamental to communication, citizenship and emotional well-being. Advocates of emotional literacy in schools argue that the skills need to be taught in

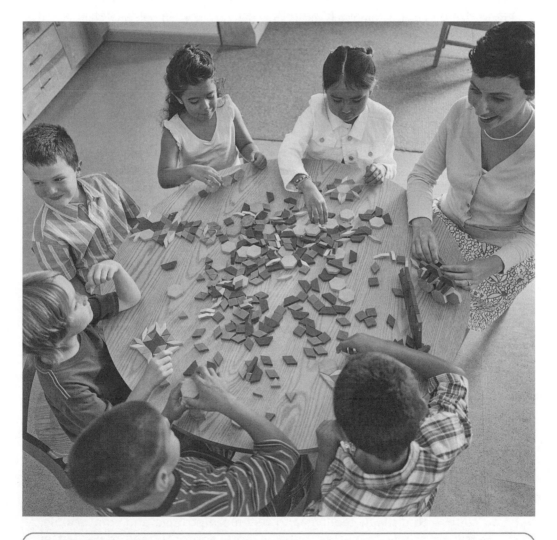

Siri Stafford/Getty images

school since, depending on their experiences in the family and the community, children vary widely in their competence in this domain. Bruce (2010) proposes that, when planning for emotional literacy, the teacher needs to consider long-term ways of creating a classroom environment that facilitates the health and well-being of all pupils. This can be achieved by thinking carefully about the quality of the relationships in the class, being sensitive to the individual needs of each young person, negotiating class contracts with the pupils and encouraging children to take responsibility for managing their own behaviour and emotions in the class community. Regular times for reflection and debriefing are an intrinsic part of the approach. This child-centred approach to learning is essentially inclusive and, when carried out with commitment, can foster democratic, respectful relationships in each class group. There is concern to meet the needs of all children, not least those who have particular social, emotional and behavioural needs. 'Circle time' will feature regularly in the emotionally literate classroom. Bruce (ibid.: 47) recommends some basic principles:

- Ensure that the circle is completely inclusive so that no one is left out; each child should be able to see every other child.
- Establish ground rules with the children about acceptable behaviour within the circle; these should refer to everyone's rights and responsibilities; everyone has the right to speak and to be heard; there should be no put downs.
- Start and end with a fun activity so that everyone feels happy, safe and confident.
- The circle should empower the children to participate with confidence, independence and ownership of their circle.

The most widely-used emotional literacy programme in the UK is Social and Emotional Aspects of Learning (SEAL) (DCSF, 2007), currently adopted in over 90% of primary schools and over 70% of secondary schools in England. The aim of SEAL is to develop five key social and emotional skills derived from research into emotional intelligence (Goleman, 1995; Salovey & Mayer, 1990). The five skills are described in Box 2.7.

Box 2.7

Definitions of the five social and emotional skills promoted through SEAL (adapted from DCSF, 2007: 5–6)

- *Self-awareness*: knowing and valuing myself and understanding how I think and feel. When we can identify and describe our beliefs, values and feelings, and feel good about ourselves, our strengths and limitations, we can learn more effectively and engage in positive interactions with others.
- *Self regulation/managing feelings*: managing how we express emotions, coping with and changing difficult and uncomfortable feelings, and increasing and enhancing positive and pleasant feelings. When we have strategies for expressing our feelings in a positive way and for helping us to cope with difficult feelings and feel more positive and comfortable, we can concentrate better, behave more appropriately, make better

relationships, and work more cooperatively and productively with those around us.

- *Motivation*: working towards goals, and being more persistent, resilient and optimistic. When we can set ourselves goals, work out effective strategies for reaching those goals, and respond effectively to setbacks and difficulties, we can approach learning situations in a positive way and maximize our ability to achieve our potential.
- *Empathy*: understanding others' thoughts and feelings and valuing and supporting others. When we can understand, respect and value other people's beliefs, values and feelings, we can be more effective in making relationships, working with and learning from people from diverse backgrounds.
- *Social skills*: building and maintaining relationships and solving problems, including interpersonal ones. When we have strategies for forming and maintaining relationships, and for solving problems and conflicts with other people, we have the skills that help us achieve all of these learning outcomes, for example, by reducing negative feelings and distraction while in learning situations, and using our interactions with others as an important way of improving our learning experience.

Unlike many of the emotional literacy programmes in the USA (e.g., Greenberg *et al.*, 2005), SEAL is not a package and schools are actively encouraged to explore different ways of delivering it depending on their specific needs. The SEAL materials are accompanied by guidance, additional resources and staff training. Emphasis is placed on building a positive school ethos, engagement of all pupils and warm personal relationships. Perhaps because of this very diversity of delivery, it has been difficult to make overall judgements about its effectiveness. Banerjee (2010) found that pupils and staff rated their school ethos more highly where SEAL was implemented according to the guidance – that is, embedded in a whole-school approach, with real support from the leadership, engagement of all staff and inclusive provision for all pupils.

The largest evaluation was carried out in primary (Humphrey *et al.*, 2008) and secondary schools (Humphrey *et al.*, 2010). In the evaluation of secondary SEAL, the research team investigated Year 7 pupils in 22 SEAL schools and a matched group of 19 comparison schools. They found, on the one hand, that pupils' feelings of autonomy and influence increased during the SEAL implementation period; they also found some improvements in behaviour, interpersonal skills and relationships. On the other hand, the research team found many barriers to the implementation of SEAL, notably lack of commitment by staff and inadequate resources. In general, they found that SEAL failed to impact on pupils' social and emotional skills, general mental health difficulties, prosocial behaviour or behaviour problems. However, in schools where there was an existing strong commitment to pastoral care combined with a high level of staff training and development, the impact of SEAL was much greater. They recommended that, in future, there should be more engagement with families/carers and a much more structured approach to the delivery of SEAL. Specifically, this research indicates that an approach that is too open-ended and flexible runs the risk that the fundamental principles will not be delivered in practice. As a result, it is not surprising that, in these circumstances, the impact is not substantial. Humphrey *et al.* (ibid.: 103) conclude that a much more rigorous structure and consistency in the actual implementation of programmes such as SEAL would ensure a stronger effect. This entails the following sequenced, active, focused and explicit (SAFE) principles to inform practice:

- *Sequenced*: the application of a planned set of activities to develop skills sequentially in a step-by-step approach;
- *Active*: the use of active forms of learning such as role play;
- *Focused*: the devotion of sufficient time exclusively to the development of social and emotional skills; and
- *Explicit*: the targeting of specific social and emotional skills.

Finally, the researchers recommend that educators learn from the successful implementation of much more structured programmes, such as the Promoting Alternative Thinking Strategies (PATHS), Second Step and Roots of Empathy.

Whereas emotional literacy programmes like SEAL target all children, some interventions focus instead on children with specific needs, such as children with social, emotional and behavioural difficulties (SEBD). Box 2.8 explores the case of children and young people with **Asperger syndrome**.

Box 2.8

Mind-reading in individuals with Asperger syndrome

Asperger syndrome affects around 1 in 200 people and is a developmental disorder that falls within the broader category of **autistic spectrum disorders (ASD)** (Baron-Cohen *et al.*, 2000). The diagnostic criteria for ASD include three fundamental impairments:

- Qualitative impairments in social interaction (for example, lack of eye-contact);
- Qualitative impairments in communication (for example, delays in language development, a lack of make-believe play);
- Restricted, repetitive and stereotyped patterns of behaviour, interests and activities (for example, inflexible adherence to specific routines and rituals).

Individuals with Asperger syndrome are often of average or above-average intelligence and are typically characterized by their intense absorption in specific topics, with a strong commitment to gaining knowledge about that topic. Consequently, it is thought that many of the most creative scientists and artists (including Leonardo da Vinci, Ludwig van Beethoven and Vincent van Gogh) have been people with Asperger syndrome. On the other hand, many have problems with social interaction and social communication, they lack empathy for others' feelings, and they often find it hard to make friends. Typically they tend not to perform well on theory of mind tasks, indicating their difficulty in understanding the mental representations of other people. Their inability to understand others' point of view means that they will take things literally and often miss the point of jokes or metaphors. Some children with Asperger syndrome have very clear ideas of right and wrong. They can become outraged if a rule is broken which poses huge problems during games with others if, as often happens, classmates cheat or invent new rules. At school, they encounter many such difficulties in everyday situations, often by misreading non-verbal cues from teachers and peers and, as a result, responding inappropriately, sometimes with angry outbursts or by withdrawing into their own private world. Failure to realize that other people have independent beliefs, makes it hard for these children and young people to interpret why others behave as they do, and this can severely hamper their effective functioning in social situations. Because they are perceived as different, they are vulnerable to being bullied and socially rejected by peers. Consequently, many have low self-esteem, feelings of loneliness and a tendency to blame others. Their isolation from the peer group can become most intense during adolescence. Case Study 2.4 indicates how important it is to intervene early to help these children.

CASE STUDY 2.4

Supporting Toby: a boy with Asperger syndrome

Toby is 8 years old and of high intelligence. He lives with his mother, Zoe, and older brother, Nathan, who is popular and outgoing, and very successful academically. His parents are divorced and he sees his Dad at weekends. School assessments are consistently high in English, Maths and Science. However, Toby also needs very clear interventions from his teacher, Miss Jahan, to support his learning. Without this support he frequently lapses into dreamlike states while he thinks deeply about one aspect of his work, such as the right word in a story, so that his work tends not to be finished. When asked by Miss Jahan, 'Why have you not finished your work?' he will typically reply, 'I'm thinking'. If Miss Jahan prompts him with questions like, 'What is your next sentence?', Toby will write very imaginative and sophisticated pieces using vocabulary far in advance of his classmates. With regard to peer relationships, Toby finds it hard to make eye contact. He finds it very difficult to deal with the frequently changing rules of games and often gets very upset in child-led activities.

Zoe is very sensitive to Toby's needs but can appear defensive when his issues are raised by the school, especially with regard to peer relationships and his difficulties in attending to academic work. However, she appreciates the school's suggestions for supporting Toby's learning and for helping him to develop social skills. The newly appointed Special Educational Needs Coordinator (SENCO), Mr Walker, had established a friendship group and proposed that Toby should join it. This small group focused on cooperative games, listening skills and the sharing of thoughts and feelings. After a term of attending the friendship group, Toby became more at ease with other children. Meanwhile, in class, Miss Jahan ensured that she or the teaching assistant regularly prompted Toby when he went into dreamlike states. Concurrently, Toby worked weekly with a learning mentor on a one-to-one basis on projects of special interest to him, such as astronomy, and on setting targets for his class work.

By the end of the year, Toby was able to complete his work to a high standard in class and was working much more independently. Socially, Toby was able to cope much better in class. Occasionally he misinterpreted situations but generally he was much more relaxed with his peers, even though he had not yet been able to make one close friend.

Discussion question

Are there any further strategies that might be used to help Toby?

There are a number of strategies that parents and professionals can use to prepare young people with Asperger syndrome for the everyday social situations that they find so challenging. They benefit from provision of extra specialist help, not only with academic subjects, but also in dealing with social situations. Gray (2000) recommends the creation of **social story books**. These are books specifically designed for the individual, with information on what people are doing, thinking or feeling, the sequence of events, the identification of significant social happenings, and a script on what to do and say. The stories can also take the form of cartoons with feelings represented by different colours. The young person can then learn the non-verbal signals that he/she finds so difficult to read. The experience of rehearsing and practising these theory of mind scripts gives the young person with Asperger syndrome increased understanding of their social world. Wellman *et al.* (2002) similarly recommend the use of **thought bubbles**. The researchers tested a 'picture-in-the-head' strategy in which thought bubbles coming out of the heads of cartoon characters portrayed 'what the person is thinking'. These included the kinds of situations that children with Asperger syndrome find especially difficult, for example, when two people have different thoughts about the same event. This teaching method was successful with at least some of the children in their sample since the strategy provided them with a technique for thinking about the mental state concepts that underlie the difficulties that these children experience in everyday social interaction and communication.

Nurture groups

This section considers the work of the nationwide Nurture Group Network. There are currently around 1,500 **nurture groups** (NGs) active in the UK. Nurture groups vary in nature depending on the settings in which they take place. The main common aspect is that they are grounded in attachment theory, an area of psychology which explains the need for any person to be able to form secure and happy relationships with others in the formative years of their lives (see Chapter 3).

There are some insecurely attached children who are already displaying social, emotional and behavioural difficulties during the pre-school years. For these children the transition to primary school can be particularly problematic. Because they cannot relate well to others, such children find it very difficult to settle in school. Many of the children who are placed in NGs have experienced disruptive or dysfunctional parenting in their early years. For this reason, they tend to have limited capacity to regulate their emotions and consequently experience acute difficulties in their relationships with peers. The rationale that underpins nurture groups is that the children have, for a number of reasons, missed out on the early experiences in the home that promote positive, trusting relationships with peers and adults. The NG teacher's role is to understand the gaps in these children's development and to try to meet their particular needs.

NGs, usually of between 6 and 8 children, have many of the features of family life, such as soft furnishings, kitchen and dining facilities, where the children can experience an environment that is predictable, secure and structured. There are always two members of staff present in an NG. The children typically spend a large part of the week in the NG, gradually joining in with mainstream activities as they become ready. The relationship with the NG teachers is supportive and these teachers provide a role model that the children observe and, over time, begin to incorporate into their own relationships. The mainstream curriculum is interspersed with programmed activities, such as free-play and physical activity. A crucial feature of the NG is 'breakfast' which usually occurs mid-morning. Pupils and teachers share in a simple cooked meal (usually toast and jam) and interact socially as they eat.

Evaluations of the impact of NGs (e.g., Bennathan & Boxall, 1998; Cooper *et al.*, 2001; Cooper & Whitebread, 2007; OFSTED, 2011) reveal significant improvements in terms of children's social and emotional development, social engagement and behaviours showing secure attachment. Most of these pupils are able to transfer the psychological and behavioural changes from the NG to the mainstream classroom and make a successful transition. Reynolds *et al.*, (2009), studying 179 pupils with SEBD aged between 5 and 7 years of age of whom half were in schools with NGs and half in mainstream provision, found that the NG pupils made significant gains in self-esteem, self-image, emotional maturity and attainment in literacy when compared with those without NGs.

Emotional difficulties have a profound impact on children's capacity to deal with everyday life. In situations where the risk is balanced by protective factors, the child or young person and their family are much more likely to demonstrate resilience, even when going through periods of instability or change. This is where the timing of appropriate support is crucial. The National Institute of Clinical Excellence (NICE) (2008, 2009a) issued guidance for promoting the well-being of children and young people at both primary and secondary levels. NICE recommended that schools adopt a whole-school approach with provision for identifying and assessing early signs of emotional distress and behavioural problems.

One example can be found in the creation of Behaviour and Educational Support Teams (BESTs) to provide programmes for groups and individuals to address the difficulties that they are experiencing within the school system. Evaluations (e.g., Halsey *et al.*, 2005) indicate improvements in attendance, behaviour, attainment and emotional health and well-being of the pupils. Additionally, staff report deeper understanding of the factors that lead to such behaviour in young people.

Chapter summary

Self-concept and emotions: in the early years, the child's sense of self is closely bound up in the relationship with significant caregivers. The responsiveness of these adults is crucial.

Awareness of self and others: the child's awareness of self as a separate entity from others emerges over time. Self-concept has different dimensions, including self-image, self-esteem and ideal self.

The early years: the precursors of empathy can be seen in the behaviour of very young babies and this evolves through the quality of relationships with significant adults. Empathy is closely related to the child's concept of self and to the child's developing theory of mind.

The primary school years: by this stage, children are developing more self-awareness and greater capacity to regulate their emotions. Self-esteem is strongly influenced by the experience with peers that the child has during the primary school years, for example in the active and social selves.

Adolescence: by the time of adolescence, there are dramatic changes in self-concept. There are many significant transitions at this stage, often accompanied by greater anxiety about self-image (including body image) as the young person experiences the physical and emotional changes of puberty, and as the influence of the peer group increases. Identity formation is a critical developmental task at this stage.

The chapter finished with a brief overview of interventions such as SEAL, designed to promote emotional literacy in children and young people. There are also examples of interventions to support young people with specific emotional and behavioural difficulties.

Discussion points

- At what age does a baby develop a sense of self?
- What are the benefits of developing a theory of mind?
- Is it possible to teach emotional literacy?

Further reading

For an excellent research-based account of what emotional literacy is and how the teacher can implement it in the nursery and primary school classroom, read: Bruce, C. (2010) *Emotional Literacy in the Early Years*, London: Sage. There are illustrative case studies and practical guidelines. See also: Joliffe, W. (2007) *Cooperative Learning in the Classroom: Putting it into Practice*, London: Sage, for a wealth of ideas on creating a cooperative classroom. A similar approach focused on children with social, emotional and behavioural difficulties is found in: Cefai, C. & Cooper, P. (2009) *Promoting Emotional Education*, London: Jessica Kingsley. For a detailed discussion of the development of identity, see J. Kroger (2004) (ed.) *Discussions on Ego-identity*, Hillsdale, NJ: Lawrence Erlbaum.

Harris, P. L. (1989) *Children and Emotion,* Oxford: Basil Blackwell, is a classic text on children's representations of self and others.

Fernyhough, C. (2008) *The Baby in the Mirror*, London: Granta, gives a perceptive account, grounded in deep knowledge of developmental psychology, of the author's growing relationship with his daughter during the first three years of her life.

Frosh, S., Phoenix, A. & Pattmen, R. (2002) *Young Masculinities*, Basingstoke: Palgrave, gives fascinating insights into the ways in which boys and young men perceive themselves, their peers, their relationships and their sense of their own masculinity.

Lawrence, C. (2010) *Successful School Change and Transition for the Child with Asperger Syndrome: A Guide for Parents*, London: Jessica Kingsley, is a guide for parents, written in a straightforward style, and full of practical suggestions for strategies that prepare the child with Asperger syndrome for changing school, for example, visiting the new school in advance, photographing and mapping routes and identifying potential difficulties.

Dowling, M. (2010) *Young Children's Personal, Social and Emotional Development*, 3rd edition, London: Sage, addresses key aspects of working with and caring for very young children and has insightful material on children's emotional and spiritual development.

Websites and resources

The Asperger Syndrome Foundation provides useful information on the nature of the syndrome and how to live with it. The Foundation also runs training seminars:
    http://www.aspergerfoundation.org.uk/what_as.htm

See also Tony Attwood's website for a wealth of information and up-to-date methods for supporting parents, professionals and people with Asperger syndrome:
    http://www.tonyattwood.com.au/

For examples of children engaged in emotional literacy lessons, including Circle Time and cooperative parachute games:
    www.sagepub.co.uk/christinebruce

European Network on Social and Emotional Competence (ENSEC) is devoted to the development and promotion of evidence-based practice in relation to socio-emotional competence and resilience among school students in Europe. It has a journal and newsletter as well as a conference:
    http://www.enseceurope.org/

The Collaborative for Academic, Social, and Emotional Learning (CASEL) aims to establish social and emotional learning as an essential part of education. The website contains a wealth of practical and research information:
    http://casel.org/

Information on the evaluation of Social and Emotional Aspects of Learning (SEAL) can be found on the website of the Department for Education:
    http://www.education.gov.uk/search/results?q=social+and+emotional+aspects+of+learning

Quality Circle Time. This model presents a whole-school approach to promoting positive relationships, creating a caring and respectful ethos and helping children develop their self-esteem and self-confidence:
    www.circle-time.co.uk/

The Nurture Group Network gives information about the nationwide network as well as reading and fascinating video material about the method in action:
www.nurturegroups.org/

Roots of Empathy is considered a model of social innovation. There are two programmes: a flagship programme called *The Roots of Empathy* and a programme for children aged 3 to 5 years in early childhood settings, called *Seeds of Empathy*:
http://www.rootsofempathy.org

Second Step is a popular programme for developing emotional literacy:
http://www.cfchildren.org/programs/ssp/overview/

Ebb and Flo is an animated series for a young audience. Ebb is a grumpy but sweet, portly dog and Flo, a little girl, is Ebb's best friend. They live with Ma on a boat. This gentle series follows Ebb and Flo as they spend their days playing around the boatyard or on the beach. Bird befriends the pair and follows Ebb around, generally getting in the way like any younger sibling. 'Grrr' says Ebb.

In the stories Ebb shows a range of emotions humans often try to hide. But Flo helps Ebb cope with each new experience as it comes along. So with Flo at Ebb's side and Bird right behind, Ebb can find a way through. In the *Ebb and Flo* DVD, the episode 'Ebb's new friend' provides opportunities to discuss friendship and the emotions that are an integral part of it.
www.ebbandflo.com

Chapter 3

Attachment

Map of the chapter

This chapter charts the development of attachment relationships between children, parents/caregivers and different family members, including siblings, grandparents and step-parents. It discusses the processes that lead to secure or insecure attachment, as well as the Strange Situation Test, and other measures of attachment. The chapter considers the impact on children of separation and loss. Links are made between theory of mind and the internal working model of relationships. Multiple attachments are considered, as well as cultural differences in the expression of attachment relationships. The chapter also explores the resilience of children who have been separated from their biological parents. The study of the English and Romanian adoptees is given as an example.

The development of attachment

Chapter 2 explored the development of the self and emphasized the critical role of the relationship between the growing child and the significant adults and peers in the child's life. The present chapter continues to examine the impact of early family relationships on the development of the child's inner world, sense of self and capacity to form meaningful bonds with others. Attachments can form at any age but the most intense study by psychologists has been that of the very first relationship that forms between baby and the primary caregiver, usually, but not always, the mother. The focus here is on **attachment theory**, as initially proposed in detail by

Bowlby (1969), grounded in his therapeutic work as a child psychiatrist and psychoanalyst. Bowlby's theory has been greatly extended and refined by his followers. Over the past 40 years, researchers and practitioners have gathered a substantial body of knowledge about the significance of the bond between parents and their children. The concept of attachment integrates social, emotional and cognitive aspects of the child's mind. As Cassidy (1999: 5) observes, 'Within this framework, attachment is considered a normal and healthy characteristic of humans throughout the lifespan, rather than a sign of immaturity that needs to be outgrown'.

Key concepts in Bowlby's (1969) original formulation of the theory are *affectional bonds*, *attachment* and *attachment behaviour*.

- An *affectional bond* is an enduring emotional tie to a specific individual. A person can be attached to someone who is not in turn attached to him or her.
- *Attachment* is a type of affectional bond characterized by physical proximity-seeking, comfort and security, separation upset and reciprocity.
- *Attachment behaviour* is any form of behaviour that results in a person attaining proximity to some other differentiated and preferred individual usually conceived as stronger and/or wiser. As such, the behaviour includes the following: clinging, crying, calling, greeting, smiling and some more sophisticated forms.

Bowlby proposed that the child uses the mother (or primary caregiver) as a secure base to return to regularly for reassurance. The need to explore takes the infant away from the caregiver and counteracts the need for proximity. A balance is struck between the two opposing tendencies – the need for proximity and the need to explore. In a situation of threat, attachment behaviours, such as clinging, will be reactivated.

Bowlby (ibid.) described the following phases in the development of attachment (Box 3.1):

Box 3.1

Four phases of attachment (adapted from Bowlby, 1969: 79)

- *Indiscriminate social responsiveness* (0–2 months): the infant orientates and signals without discriminating between different people.
- *Attachment to familiar people* (3–7 months): the infant shows preference to one or more discriminated persons and is more responsive to familiar caregivers. This is the beginning of attachment. The infant is more likely to smile at parents or to be comforted by parents when distressed.
- *Intense attachments* (8 months onwards): the infant maintains proximity to a preferred person by means of locomotion and signals. For example, the infant crawls after the person or returns regularly for contact, or cries if the person leaves. This stage marks the onset of intense attachment to parents or caregivers. One related phenomenon is that the infant becomes wary of strangers.
- *Goal-corrected attachment* (24 months onwards): goal-corrected partner-ships – two-sided relationships – occur between the child and the caregiver.

Up to this point, the parents have served as a resource for the child, available when needed. From around 2 years onwards, the child begins to accommodate to the parents' needs, by delaying his/her own plans and goals, for example, by waiting until the parent returns rather than crying inconsolably.

Discussion question

Bowlby referred mainly to the mother as primary caregiver and was criticized for this emphasis, particularly when he wrote about maternal deprivation. Discuss how the role of primary caregiver might vary between cultures.

Security of attachment and the internal working model of relationships

As the child's social world expands, so the need for proximity to the primary caregivers lessens. Cassidy (1999: 5) notes that the flexible use of a variety of attachment behaviours, adapted to the circumstances, gives the child greater efficiency in goal-corrected responses. In other words, children develop a range of attachment styles that ensure survival in different emotional climates. Children also develop the ability to think about attachment relationships, even when the primary caregivers are not there. According to Bowlby, this is the beginning of the **internal working model of relationships (IWM)**. By this, he meant the cognitive structures that embody the memories of day-to-day interactions with the primary caregiver. These 'event scripts' guide the child's actions and expectations with the attachment figure, based on previous interactions. In other words, the child is forming a sense of the relationship that does not only rely on physical proximity but rather on qualities, such as affection, trust and feelings of being valued. These memories or cognitions of the relationship guide the child's actions and emotions based on previous experience with the parent and future expectations of the relationship. It is possible to get a sense of the child's internal working model by listening to their narratives as they play or by observing how they respond to new experiences or people.

Bowlby's ideas on affectional bonds were greatly refined by Ainsworth *et al.* (1978) who investigated in more detail the nature of the secure base and the variety of parenting styles that children experienced in different contexts. (Ainsworth's early work was with mothers and babies in rural Uganda and in urban USA.) She is famous for designing the Strange Situation Test (Box 3.2). Following Bowlby's theory, she had observed that, at around the age of 8 months, even in widely contrasting cultures, babies typically became wary of strangers and would seek out their attachment figure (usually the mother) when under this perceived threat. Ainsworth's test was designed to investigate the fear of strangers more deeply. The experiment, lasting for about 20 minutes, involves seven short episodes which take place in the following sequence as shown in Box 3.2; the episodes are filmed for further analysis:

Box 3.2

The Strange Situation Test (Ainsworth *et al.*, 1978)

1 A mother and her baby play together in a pleasant room with attractive toys and surroundings (around 3 minutes);
2 Then a stranger (usually a young researcher who is experienced in relating well to young children) comes into the room and sits (1 minute); she talks to the mother (1 minute) and tries to interact with the baby (around 1 minute);
3 Then, at a signal, the mother leaves the room unobtrusively while the baby is engrossed with a toy; the stranger continues to interact with the baby (3 minutes);
4 The mother returns and the stranger leaves the room; the mother comforts the baby (3 minutes);
5 The mother then leaves the room again, leaving the baby alone (up to 3 minutes);
6 The stranger comes in and tries to settle the baby then withdraws, if possible (up to 3 minutes);
7 Finally, the mother returns and the stranger leaves the room. The mother comforts the child and they play together.

Discussion question

Why were there such differences in the behaviour of the baby when separated from his/her mother?

Ainsworth observed that babies reacted to this situation in different ways. Some cried when their mothers left but were quickly comforted on reunion. Others seemed to be indifferent as to whether the mother was present or absent. Others were very preoccupied and clingy with their mothers both before and after the separation. Securely attached babies, it was predicted, would use the mother as a secure base in order to explore the toys and other attractive things in the environment (episodes 1, 2 and 4) but would be distressed by the mother's absence (episodes 3, 5 and 6). Ainsworth and her team paid special attention to the points of reunion to observe how easily the baby was comforted by the mother (episodes 4 and 7). On the basis of their analysis of the infants' behaviour in the different episodes, Ainsworth and her colleagues identified three main types of attachment. Later, Main and Hesse (1990) identified a fourth category which is also included here (see Box 3.3).

Box 3.3

Four types of attachment (adapted from Ainsworth *et al.*, 1978; Main & Hesse, 1990)

- *Insecurely attached: detached/avoidant (Type A)*: The child focuses on toys or the environment throughout the experiment; does not cry on separation from the parent. The child avoids contact with the mother on reunion, or shows avoidance responses, such as turning away, moving past or averting gaze; does not resist contact but shows no preference for the mother in preference to the stranger. The response to the parent on reunion appears unemotional. During separations, such children do not appear to be distressed.
- *Securely attached (Type B)*: The child is happy to explore the environment but returns to the mother when upset; shows signs of missing the parent during separation but is easily comforted on reunion; greets the mother actively on her return, usually initiating physical contact. Securely attached children are characterized by actively seeking and maintaining proximity, contact or interaction with the primary caregiver. They show obvious preference for the parent over the stranger.
- *Insecurely attached: resistant/ambivalent (Type C)*: The child appears preoccupied with the parent throughout the experiment; may seem angry or passive. The child is not so happy to explore the environment and may be wary even prior to separation; is very upset on separation from mother and is difficult to comfort on reunion; both seeks and resists comfort – hence the term 'resistant/ambivalent'. After the reunion, fails to explore the toys or the environment.
- *Insecurely attached: disorganized/disoriented (Type D):* The child displays disorganized and/or disoriented behaviours in the parent's presence. For example, the child may freeze with a trance-like expression, hands in the air. After separation, the child appears to seek comfort while avoiding gaze, or expresses distress, or is ambivalent. Their responses are inconsistent and bizarre.

Discussion question

Describe some of the behaviours that you have observed in everyday situations, for example, when collecting a child from day care or while babysitting. Explain them in the light of this classification.

Box 3.3 shows the main attachment types, each of which has a number of sub-categories. Type B babies (secure) are in the majority, and secure attachment is viewed by Ainsworth *et al.* (1978) as the more advantageous condition for the infant in comparison with Types A and C and (later) D (insecure). One explanation for the different attachment types was suggested by Ainsworth and her team. They proposed that the quality of the mother-baby relationship predicted secure or insecure attachment.

More recent research confirms this view by arguing that parents' mind-mindedness is an important influence (Meins *et al.*, 2002) (as discussed in Chapter 2). Many studies indicate that the presence of secure or insecure attachment in infancy has a strong influence over the quality of relationships throughout childhood, both in the family and at day care and school. A critical aspect concerns the different internal working models of securely and insecurely attached children. As discussed earlier in this chapter, secure attachment (Type B) would be represented by constructions of trust, affection and openness about emotions; the securely attached child appears to have a mental representation of the attachment figure as available and responsive when needed. Insecurely attached children would differ. The insecure avoidant child (Type A) would be likely to have an internal working model tending towards mistrust and with little expectation of comfort when in distress. This would be accompanied by a less open form of communication. An insecure resistant child (Type C), by contrast, would have an internal working model characterized by ambivalence and uncertainty about what to expect.

As Main and Solomon (1990) argue, in comparison to the insecurely attached (Types A and C), the prediction for later childhood would be that securely attached children (Type B) would be more likely to:

● have positive relationships with their peers;
● have more friends and be more confident with adults;
● have higher self-esteem;
● be less likely to have emotional and behavioural difficulties;
● be more confident during adolescence;
● have more satisfying romantic relationships as adults.

One longitudinal study (Kochanska, 2001) followed up children from 9 to 33 months old and found that, over time, the Type A babies became more fearful, Type C babies became less joyful and Type D babies became more angry; by contrast, Type B babies showed less fear, anger and distress. Kochanska concluded that the mutually cooperative orientation facilitated by a secure parent-infant attachment promotes many positive aspects of psychosocial growth, including theory of mind and autobiographical memories.

However, Crittenden (1995) criticizes the choice of labels 'secure' and 'insecure' on the grounds that they imply that Type A and Type C children are disturbed. This, she argues, is not necessarily the case. From Crittenden's perspective, attachment patterns reflect a dynamic balance between reliance on affective and cognitive processes. Type A individuals direct more attention and energy to cognitive activities and only minimal attention to emotion-laden relationships. Type C children are more focused on emotional relationships to the exclusion of intellectual activities. (In any case, these are the extremes, with many individuals at different points along the continuum.) The different patterns represent a form of adaptation to a particular family or cultural method of child-rearing.

Nevertheless, the Type D children are at much greater risk of developing attachment disorders, as indicated by Amy in Case Study 3.1. The Type D pattern is evident when primary caregivers are highly abusive, depressed or emotionally disturbed. These children have experienced some form of traumatic separation from the primary caregiver, or have experienced severe neglect and abuse. They appear to be preoccupied with unresolved processes of mourning over the loss of their primary attachment figure (Crittenden, 1988). Crittenden (1992) considers that even the disorganized Type D infants are displaying a form of adaptation to the constraints of the abusive or neglectful situation in which they find themselves. She prefers to call this pattern *defended/coercive* rather than *disorganized* as she views the infant's behaviour as strategic rather than passive.

CASE STUDY 3.1

Amy: a looked-after child

Amy was born when her mother, Hazel, was 18 years old. Hazel had had a very insecure childhood and was addicted to drugs and alcohol. Soon after the birth, Hazel's 19-year-old boyfriend left after a stormy and violent disagreement. Hazel had no stable family to turn to and sought security from multiple partners. Social services were alerted by neighbours because Amy was often left alone in the house while Hazel was out with boyfriends. By the time she was 4 years old, Amy was taken into foster care because of extreme neglect. By this time, Amy's behaviour was unmanageable at home and at nursery. The foster mother found Amy extremely difficult and the placement broke down after 6 months.

Social services sought one of their most experienced foster parents, Jane. During this placement, it came to light that not only had Amy suffered physical neglect but also sexual abuse at the hands of a babysitter. Masturbation in public was one of a range of behaviours that Amy demonstrated. To her, it was only a form of self-soothing. Jane understood why Amy did this but when she discovered Amy encouraging a younger child in her family to engage in mutual masturbation, she felt that she could no longer continue as foster parent. It was realized that Amy needed to be in a placement with no other children.

The social worker found an appropriate placement with Brian and Eve, an older couple whose own children were grown up. They were professional foster parents, in that they had done accredited training on attachment disorders as well as on child development. The foster parents are well supported by social services, who provide continuing training in attachment disorders in adolescence, by a dedicated social worker, as well as through their own personal skills as foster parents. This placement has been successful and is into its tenth year.

There have been many difficulties. Amy's behaviour included frequent temper tantrums, trashing her bedroom, breaking toys and electronic devices. She had poor personal hygiene and often refused to wash. She could not always control her habit of masturbating while watching TV. But Eve persisted in accepting Amy. She bought her special soap and shower gel. She explained calmly and non-judgementally why it is important not to masturbate in public. Eve knew that she would always have to be alert to Amy's difficult behaviours and work with her on a daily basis to help her manage them. Eve continued to view this reassurance as part of her role as a professional foster parent.

To date, Amy does not have close friends. Her peers at school find her strange but they tolerate her and show kindness and understanding for the most part. In her school, peer support is actively encouraged. The school has peer mentors who ensure that Amy is not on her own at break times and lunchtimes. Amy is now doing well at secondary school. She is learning to manage her own needs and understands that some behaviours are socially unacceptable. At school, she has discovered a talent for dance and drama which she really enjoys. This brings her a feeling of success and achievement. Throughout, despite Amy's challenging behaviour, the foster parents, Brian and Eve, demonstrated their belief in her, supported by the social worker and other agencies. Their resilience provided Amy with the secure base she so desperately needed.

Discussion questions

If you were interviewing people who had applied to be foster parents what are the qualities that you would be looking for? What sustained Brian and Eve during the most difficult times with Amy? How important is multi-agency team work for supporting foster parents?

In working with looked-after children like Amy, social workers and foster parents have learned so much. Children like Amy teach us how to help other children who have been neglected or abused. Case studies like this, however disturbing, help professionals and potential foster parents to understand the children in their care more deeply.

Attachment beyond infancy

Multiple attachments

The majority of children become attached to more than one familiar person during their first year, typically siblings, grandparents, aunt and uncles, but in some cultures there will also be a wide extended family network (Ainsworth, 1967). Although children have multiple attachment figures, they will not treat them all in the same way. Bowlby (1969: 304) acknowledged that most infants form more than one attachment, for example, to siblings, grandparents, aunts and uncles: 'almost from the first, many children have more than one figure to whom they direct attachment behaviour'. However, this number is not limitless. The infant will typically not treat all attachment figures in the same way, as if they were interchangeable, but will show preference for one or two primary caregivers, particularly when in a situation where the infant is distressed. Looked-after children will, if given the opportunity, select one special caregiver as their own

(Cassidy, 1999: 14). By middle childhood, opportunities for new attachments arise at school and in the community. By adolescence and young adulthood, relationships with romantic and sexual partners become increasingly central.

A number of researchers have pointed to the huge impact that siblings have on children's and adolescents' lives as significant role models. Around 80% of children grow up in families with at least one brother or sister. Usually they differ in age by at least a year and typically two or three years. Interactions between siblings help to facilitate the development of theory of mind, that is, the ability to understand the thoughts and emotions of other people. This understanding seems to grow through the multiple, everyday interactions with siblings, for example, when they engage in extensive pretend-play which involves negotiation about internal emotional states and motivation for action. There is strong evidence that having a sibling can accelerate the development of theory of mind development in the under-fives. Older siblings are often very tolerant of their younger siblings but, at the same time, they can also show hostility. The inevitable conflicts with siblings offer potential for learning about fairness, moral rules about property, turn-taking and sharing. The nature of these experiences – for example, aggressive or cooperative – can have far-reaching effects. Dunn *et al.* (1991) found that in early adolescence, someone who had grown up with an unfriendly or hostile sibling was more likely to be anxious, depressed or aggressive. Where the child has no siblings, similar processes can of course take place through interactions with family members. But there is something very special about the relationship with a sibling. There is also evidence to show that only children, once they reach school age, are more likely to be nominated by their peers as aggressive or withdrawn and are more likely to be victimized by peers (Kitzmann *et al.*, 2002). One explanation is that the everyday experience of negotiating with a near-age sibling is a great

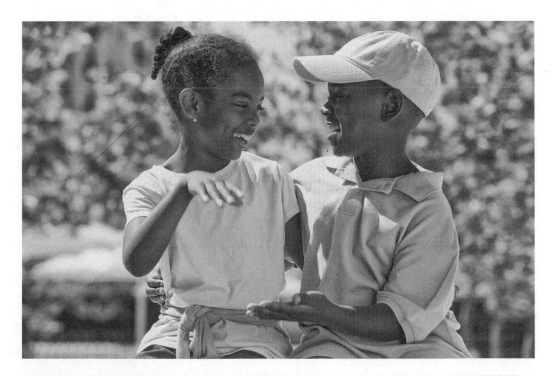

BLOOM image/Getty images

preparation for the rough and tumble of relationships with peers. Other research shows that only children get more attention from their parents and this quality time has a positive effect on their achievement.

There are many different types of stepfamily arrangement so it is difficult to make generalizations here but there is evidence that children in stepfamilies, when compared with children in intact families, typically experience a greater number of adjustment difficulties. However, the evidence is that these differences are not large and that in most cases the differences disappear over time. Adjusting to life in a new family, possibly with new stepsiblings is understandably a

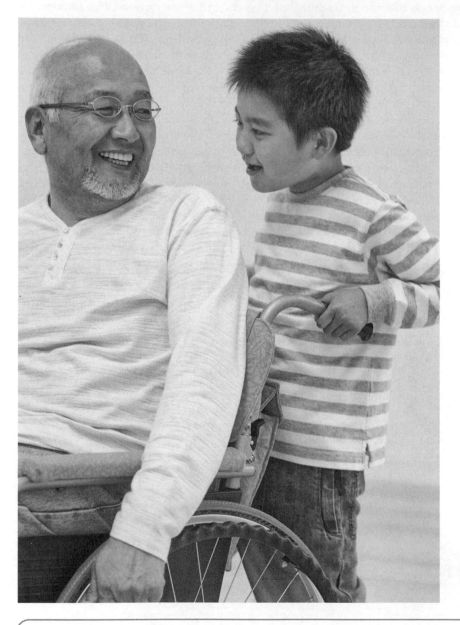

Jupiter images/Getty images

challenge but the difficulties are mediated by such factors as the quality of the relationships among the adults involved, the commitment of the step-parents to making the new relationships work and the nature of the relationships amongst the siblings and stepsiblings.

Grandparents can be very important people in the child's social network (Sear & Mace, 2007). In contemporary society they tend to provide emotional support rather than authority and discipline, and they can hand down stories from family history and information about significant historical events in society. Where there is disharmony in the child's family, for example, through marital separation and divorce, grandparents can play a critical role in supporting the child emotionally and in providing everyday care. Research indicates that relationships are less satisfying where grandparents are perceived as uninvolved with their grandchildren (not interested in babysitting, for example) or over-involved (interfering in matters of discipline).

Cultural differences

A number of cross-cultural studies have found that, across cultures, experts' conceptualizations of attachment were very similar to those of mothers. Posada *et al.* (1995), for example, in a major cross-cultural study in China, Japan, Israel, Columbia, Germany, Norway and the USA, used the Attachment Q-sort – a method for assessing the quality of a child's secure-base behaviour in the naturalistic setting of the home. Secure-base behaviour was defined as the smooth organization and appropriate balance between proximity-seeking and exploration. The researchers found close agreement between trained observers and mothers in discriminating between attachment security and other behaviours, such as dependency and social desirability. There is a wealth of evidence to support the view that the early years lay a strong foundation for later emotional security and that many of the difficulties experienced by children and young people later on can be traced back to the first relationships with primary caregivers. In all societies, primary attachments are usually with the mother, though multiple attachments exist to a greater or lesser extent in the wider family network and in the community. Parents of secure babies tend to be attentive and available across cultures. Parents of avoidant infants tend not to respond sensitively to the child's cries and signals of distress, while ambivalently attached infants are more likely to have parents who respond inconsistently.

However, there are many ways in which the attachment relationship is expressed, depending on the values and customs of the cultural group to which the child belongs. For example, Kermoian and Leiderman (1986) indicate that Gusii infants are accustomed to being greeted with a handshake instead of a hug by their parents after separation, whereas Western infants expect more intimate physical contact. Parents in different cultures value the child's security in different ways and for different reasons. Van IJzendoorn and Sagi (1999: 727) argue, on the basis of their analysis of a range of cross-cultural studies in China, Japan, Israel and Africa, that it is essential to be sensitive to the wider social networks within which children grow and develop. If researchers only rely on the mother-infant relationship, they will lack the deeper understanding of the complex factors that lead to social and emotional competence. Researchers have found quite wide cultural differences in babies' responses to the Strange Situation, suggesting that different patterns of child-rearing have a strong impact (Van IJzendoorn & Kroonenberg, 1988). For example, Takahashi (1986) urges caution when interpreting the extremely distressed reactions of Japanese children when the mother leaves the room in the Strange Situation since in Japanese families babies are never left by themselves. In order to understand more fully the dynamics of family relationships across cultures, it is necessary to be sensitive to norms and rules which are 'part of a larger web of cultural meanings regarding conceptions of self and other' (Harwood *et al.*, 1995: 141) and take account of the interplay between experience of self and understanding of the behaviour of others, with the internal working model of relationships acting as a mediator between self and culture. In the cross-cultural study by Harwood *et al.* (ibid.) the Anglo-American mothers favoured independence and autonomy in their children, whereas the Puerto Rican mothers encouraged 'proper demeanour', by which they meant respect for adults, calmness and politeness.

Resilience in the face of adversity

The children of Kauai: a longitudinal study

Researchers point to the resilience displayed by some infants and children in the face of extremely insensitive or inadequate parenting or in situations where, because of illness, the parent is unable to offer the nurturing that the baby needs. Werner and Smith (1982) carried out a longitudinal study of a cohort of infants born in the same week in 1955 on the Hawaiian island of Kauai. Most of the children grew up in supportive families. But some experienced material disadvantage and emotional neglect from their parents for a variety of reasons. Of those high-risk children, a subset, against all the odds, developed into secure, happy adolescents and competent young adults. Some protection came from these children's easygoing temperament. But most importantly, even though their parents were not able to care for them adequately, these children had experienced nurturing from significant adults, such as grandparents, older siblings, aunts, uncles or babysitters. These resilient children were skilled at turning to teachers or neighbours for comfort, approval and affirmation. School often became a place of refuge from the chaotic lifestyles at home. Such findings highlight the flexibility of attachment behaviours as a form of coping in different emotional environments. With the help of their support networks, these resilient children developed positive beliefs in themselves and feelings of competence and optimism.

The English and Romanian adoptees

As indicated earlier, Crittenden (1988) regards even insecure attachment as a strategy for coping in which, for example, avoidant or ambivalent attachment behaviours might act as a form of protection for the infant. The study of the Romanian adoptees also provides crucial information about the capacity of children and adoptive families to overcome the negative effects of extremely deprived experiences in the early years (Box 3.4).

Box 3.4

The case of the English and Romanian adoptees (ERA) (adapted from Rutter *et al.*, 2009)

Michael Rutter and his colleagues carried out a unique longitudinal study of the deficit and developmental 'catch-up' of children who had spent the first years of their lives in Romanian orphanages where neglect and deprivation were the norm. These children were severely delayed by the time they came to the UK where they were adopted by loving and supportive families. They

---

were compared with a sample of UK children who had been placed for adoption before the age of 6 months. Both groups of children were assessed at the ages of 4, 6, 11 and 15 years and at young adulthood. Initial measurements at 4 years indicated great resilience on the part of the Romanian children. In particular, those who had been adopted before the age of 6 months indicated almost complete catch-up with regard to physical and cognitive development by the age of 4 years. They also appeared to show extraordinary emotional resilience. However, the outcomes for those who were adopted between the ages of 6 and 24 months were less favourable. The latest-placed children (adopted between the ages of 24 and 42 months) had long-term difficulties. The early deprivation continued to have an adverse effect on their emotional development. They were more likely to be wary of strangers and to have difficulties in their relationships with adults and their peer group, for example, by being bullied by classmates. They were also more likely to display hyperactivity and attention deficit and hyperactivity disorder (ADHD). Some of these difficulties persisted beyond the age of 11 years. The follow-up at age 15 indicated some continuation of emotional and social difficulties. On the other hand, for most of the young people in the sample there were great improvements over time. As adolescents, most of the adoptees were extremely positive about their experiences within the families. By the age of 15, around a quarter of the young people had visited Romania and valued this opportunity to discover more about their country of origin. Rutter and colleagues concluded that, if children are rescued from extreme adversity before the age of 6 months and placed in loving families, there is every chance that they will catch up. For those who are adopted after 6 months of age, there is increased risk of difficulties, especially in the domain of relationships. But even then, though some impairment seems likely to persist, it is important to allow time for improvement to take place and to provide educational and therapeutic support in the process.

Discussion question

Discuss the impact of the ERA study on the understanding of attachment relationships.

Helping children deal with separation and loss

Infants are strongly affected when they are separated from the attachment figure. When the attachment figure is inaccessible or absent, the child will attempt to re-establish contact by calling, searching and clinging, as many parents observe when they leave a young child at nursery for the first time. Prolonged separation from parents causes acute distress in infants, as James and Joyce Robertson showed in their disturbing films of young children placed temporarily in residential care (for example, when the mother was in hospital giving birth to another baby) (Robertson, 1971). The children initially cried and would not be comforted but, if the separation was prolonged, the protests and distress gave way to despair, sadness and withdrawal. A typical sequence of behaviour was as follows:

- *Distress*: protest and crying; refuses to be comforted by others.
- *Despair*: child becomes quiet and apathetic; little protest; child appears to be in a state of hopelessness.
- *Detachment*: child appears to have come to terms with separation from the parent; begins to form new relationships; on the return of the parents the child may become very clingy or very cold. Appears unable to trust the parent on return. Becomes clingy and refuses to let the parent leave in any situation.

Later the Robertsons showed that these reactions to separation from the parent could be alleviated if a trusted adult visited often, or stayed in the residential placement. In other words, if it was acknowledged that the child's grief was an understandable response, it was much easier to help the children deal with their feelings.

In each generation, a proportion of children will suffer loss of a parent, perhaps through divorce, serious illness or death. Family members and other adults involved with the child will often find that, understandably, the child's behaviour changes during such a difficult period. While many children show resilience and the capacity to cope with loss, it is essential to be aware of the huge emotional impact that separation from a loved one has on the child. The majority of children in such a situation do not receive professional help but that does not mean that they do not need support from those around them. Children who experience the loss of a parent or other significant person in their lives will need time to go through a period of mourning, just as adults do. Parkes (1972) identified certain phases that children typically go through when they are grieving:

- An initial numb phase where emotions are blunted. This can last from a few hours to two weeks or more;
- A mourning phase, characterized by intense distress, sadness, irritability and preoccupation with the person who has died, feelings of guilt or denial. Some children have hallucinatory experiences, such as imagining that they see or hear the dead person;
- Acceptance and readjustment, several weeks or more after the onset of mourning.

Parkes (ibid.) indicated that there are wide variations in the responses of children and young people to a serious loss, such as sleeplessness, calling or searching for the loved one, crying, repeatedly recalling the image of the attachment figure, experiencing helplessness, fear and despair. Children and adolescents can develop regressive behaviour. Small children, for example, may start wetting the bed, while adolescents may behave more childishly for a time. Some children isolate themselves because of lack of understanding, or even bullying, from the peer group. The duration of the process can vary according to the young person's family values and culture, and those who are unable to resolve their grief may develop atypical mourning such as:

- Chronic grief that can turn into depression;
- Delayed grief where the child or young person is slow to express their mourning or is unable to show their grief;
- Mixed reactions resulting in physical or mental health difficulties.

Dyregrov (1990) observed gender differences in children's capacity to express their feelings following bereavement. She found that boys, more than girls, tended to avoid talking about their loss, and this difference became more pronounced in adolescence. Girls in general were more likely to share feelings with a close friend and appeared to have a more developed language of emotions. The key message is that adults need to be aware of the different reactions that children will display, including psychological and physical symptoms, following a prolonged separation from, or loss of, a loved one. Adults must be aware that bereaved young people need to go through a period of mourning. One of the most helpful responses on the part of adults is to listen to the young person in whatever form – verbal or non-verbal – that their expression of emotion takes. The adult needs to demonstrate care and concern and to give time and space. Children's questions must be answered as honestly as possible. Euphemisms such as 'You have lost your mother' are less helpful that factual information. It is also important for the young person to participate in the family's mourning and to have their own unique, meaningful ceremonies, including such activities as devising a special ritual or commemoration. They also need the ongoing support of a trusted adult and the reassurance of everyday routines. If there is a risk of bullying, they need to be protected by teaching staff at school and, where these exist, by peer supporters.

Attachment across the lifespan

Whereas Ainsworth focused on the security of attachment in infancy, research by Main and Cassidy (1988) extended the measurement of attachment across the lifespan and focused more on the capacity of the child or young person to develop internal representations of relationships which would endure through to adulthood. Their work built on Bowlby's (1988) concept of the IWM (see p. 37) with significant attachment figures. Main *et al.* (1985) developed the Adult Attachment Interview in which they aimed to measure attachment in adolescence and adulthood by asking open-ended questions about the person's early childhood experiences. The transcripts were coded on the basis of the coherence of the narrative and on the capacity of the interviewee to reflect on the past. Main *et al.* (ibid.) identified four main patterns of attachment (Box 3.5):

Box 3.5

Patterns of attachment in adult life (adapted from Main *et al.*, 1985)

- *Autonomous*: people who can recall their own earlier attachment-related experiences objectively and openly, even if these were not favourable;
- *Dismissive*: people who dismiss attachment relationships as of little importance;
- *Enmeshed*: people who are preoccupied with and dependent on their own parents and still struggle to please them;
- *Unresolved*: people who have experienced trauma, or the early death of a parent, and who have not come to terms with this or been able to mourn properly.

> ### Discussion question
>
> Reflect on the correspondence between these adult patterns of attachment and the attachment types A, B, C and D of infancy. Discuss in the light of Crittenden's concept of insecure attachment as a coping strategy.

As adults, those who were detached/avoidant as infants are more likely to have difficulty with intimate adult relationships and to avoid closeness and appear unaffected when they are rejected. They may find it difficult to talk about their childhood or, alternatively, they may idealize their parents yet be unable to think of any examples to confirm this perception. With regard to children who were resistant/ambivalent, as adults they are more likely to be trapped by the unresolved struggles with the parents in ways that make it difficult for them to break free from the family. The issues from their past can overshadow adult relationships. In adulthood, the unresolved pattern is expressed through mourning over the loss of the attachment figure or the loss of childhood. These adults may be so preoccupied with unresolved issues from their early childhood that they find it difficult to meet the needs of their own children.

Disorganized/disoriented infants (Type D) are most at risk of difficulties during childhood, adolescence and adult life. Their coping strategies for dealing with unpredictable, abusive or neglectful parents have only been effective for avoiding danger rather than for having their attachment needs met. These children as they grow older are more likely to become controlling individuals, since their world is dangerous and unpredictable. In the absence of alternative attachment figures, their way of relating to others in adolescence and adulthood may be expressed through bullying and aggression, excessive control or compulsive caregiving.

Fortunately, the studies on resilience, such as the one by Werner and Smith (1982) indicate that the internal working model of relationships can be adjusted and changed in adolescence and adulthood, despite lack of a nurturing environment in infancy, if the right support networks are put in place. The inner changes in the child and young person, they argue, take place as a result of a process of reflection, from the experience of counselling or psychotherapy, by the supportive presence of an alternative attachment figure who meets the child's emotional needs in other ways, or by forming a deep relationship with an intimate friend or romantic partner. For younger children, it is likely that they need face-to-face encounters with sensitive, supportive adults. For adolescents and adults, the process can be achieved through reflections on the reasons for the lack of nurturing in early life (Case Study 3.2).

Mary: an insecurely attached person

Mary's experience of being parented was a very negative one. Beth, her mother, a single parent, suffered from post-natal depression and was not able to look after Mary in the very early years, leaving much of the day-by-day care to her own mother. Although Beth seemed to recover, the depression returned at regular intervals throughout Mary's childhood. As a result, Mary became rather with-drawn and sad and often felt very lonely. She spent a great deal of time with her grandmother who was warm and supportive. But her grandmother was also very protective of Beth and strongly discouraged any expressions of emotion on Mary's part that might distress Beth. At secondary school, Mary valued the sensitivity of her English teacher, who encouraged her to follow her interest in literature and to write her own imaginative stories, including some that expressed very angry feelings. The grandmother died when Mary was a young adult and the bereavement hit her very hard. She feared that she was going to become depressed like her mother and so she sought counselling. There she was given a safe space in which to reflect on her feelings of loss and abandonment. She also took this time to explore her feelings about her mother and the frequent absences, both physical and psychological, which had been characteristic of Mary's childhood. At this time, she was able to get in touch with her anger towards her mother, an emotion which it had always been difficult to express for fear of upsetting Beth. She also remembered occasions when Beth had told her how much she loved her. Through counselling, Mary was able to re-experience her much earlier feelings of loss which had returned on the death of her grandmother. She was also able to explore the idea that her mother loved her though she could not always be with her. This therapeutic experience enabled Mary to understand both why her mother could not always be there for her and why she herself had so often felt unhappy as a child. She was empowered to share some of these thoughts and feelings with her mother, without fearing the emotional consequences, as she had as a child. This became a form of reunion and reconciliation. As an adult, Mary was able to reframe her internal working model and move on with her life.

Discussion question

Explore the risk and protective factors in Mary's childhood. Discuss how useful attachment theory is in understanding the processes of change in Mary as an adult.

Theory of mind and the internal working model of relationships

As indicated in Chapter 2, there is a great deal of interest in the concept of the child's theory of mind, with recent attempts to integrate its cognitive and emotional aspects. Fonagy *et al.* (1997) argued that mind-reading appears early in the child's life in the context of the intense emotional relationship between infant and caregiver. Similarly, research by Dunn *et al.* (1991) showed that family interactions at 33 months of age with siblings that were characterized by diversity of emotion, discussions of cause and effect and explanations of disputed feelings, predicted higher performance at 6 years on a perspective-taking task. In other words, in families where children are given wide experience of mind-reading and encouraged to take the point of view of others (as happens in everyday life through cooperation and conflict resolution with siblings) the children are likely to have a more developed theory of mind. Box 3.6 presents some findings that support the idea of overlap between the concepts of theory of mind and the internal working model of relationships.

Box 3.6

Do the concepts of the internal working model and theory of mind overlap? (Adapted from Fonagy *et al.*, 1997)

Fonagy *et al.* (1991) collected Adult Attachment Interview material from 100 couples before the birth of their first child. They found that the frequency of these parents' references to mental states in their own childhood predicted the likelihood of secure attachment to their babies at one year (mother) and 18 months (father) in terms of the infants' response to the Strange Situation Test. They also investigated the extent of the deprivation and disrupted parenting that these adults had experienced to see if this influenced the attachment patterns of their babies. There was a trend but it was not straightforward, since there was also a strong effect from the ways in which these adults had *reflected on* their own earlier experiences. To explore this further, Fonagy *et al.* (1997) developed a scale from the Adult Attachment Interview responses – the Reflective Self-Function Scale – to measure the capacity that these parents had to reflect on their own psychological processes and emotions. Of 17 mothers with deprived parenting and low scores on the Reflective Self-Function Scale, 16 had insecurely attached infants, as measured by the Strange Situation Test. However, of 10 mothers who had similarly negative experiences as children but who scored highly on the Reflective Self-Function Scale, all had securely attached infants. These findings indicated the power of people to change their internal working model and to show resilience despite emotional hardship in the early years.

Steele *et al.* (1996) did further testing of this sample of first-born children on theory of mind tasks at 5½ years. Again, the securely attached children (Type B) were significantly more likely to perform well on theory of mind tasks than insecurely attached children, with the avoidant children (Type A) particularly likely to be unsuccessful. One interesting explanation for these findings proposed by Fonagy *et al.* (1997) is that securely attached children engage extensively in pretend-play where there is the opportunity to enter into the world of others through use of the imagination, so speculating on what goes on in the minds of others. Where the parents have the quality of **mind-mindedness** (see Chapter 2) the child is more likely to experience a safe emotional environment reflected in the caregiver's perception of the child as a person with feelings and intentions.

Discussion questions

Why did the insecurely attached children perform less well on theory of mind tasks? Why did Fonagy and colleagues consider that the insecurely attached children were less likely to engage in imaginative play? Give some examples of ways in which the process of mind-mindedness might work?

Risk and protective factors

Attachment theory demonstrates the need to take account of the quality of the interpersonal relationships within the family with regard to the emotional development of children and young people. There is greater understanding that children's behaviour – such as angry, disruptive behaviour or withdrawal from social interaction – may have its origins in attachment issues in the early years. (See, for example, the work of the Nurture Group Network, as described in Chapter 2.) There is also a growing body of evidence that children and young people play an active role in shaping their experiences, processing these experiences and giving them meaning (Meins *et al.*, 2002). There is growing recognition that there are protective mechanisms, both within the individual and in the interactions between that young person and their social and emotional environments, that can change negative experiences for the better. The influences from primary caregivers are crucial but they can be mediated by peers, siblings, grandparents and other significant people in the community.

As the child broadens the range of experiences within the family, at school and out into the community, it is important to be aware of the balance between risk and protective factors in the child's environment.

Risk factors for child development

- Family: abusive or neglectful; discordant relationships; parental mental illness; criminality; unclear disciplinary practices; lack of boundaries;
- Society: high levels of poverty and deprivation; experiences of discrimination; homelessness; being a member of a deviant group;
- Child: has chronic illness; hyperactivity; misuse of drugs or alcohol.

Protective factors for child development

- Family: good relationships; moderate family size; adequate income; clear consistent discipline; support for child's education; has a religious or moral belief system.
- Society: access to good education; a wider support network for the family; range of childcare facilities is available; liaison between school and wider community.
- Child: has sense of mastery; participates in sports, music and other activities; member of non-deviant groups; has good health; has an even temperament; has positive self-esteem and good social skills.

Chapter summary

This chapter examines the crucial role of relationships within the family for the healthy emotional and social development of the child. The relationship with the mother is usually the central one but other family members, such as foster parents, siblings and grandparents, have a significant influence too. Cross-cultural differences in the expression of attachment relationships are considered. The concept of the internal working model of relationships is proposed as an important explanation for mediating processes within the child and young person. The study of the English and Romanian adoptees indicates evidence of resilience on the part of children and young people despite extreme deprivation and neglect in the early years, and provides indicators of key protective factors.

Discussion points

- How do primary caregivers meet infants' emotional needs and why is this crucial for later relationships?
- What is the internal working model of relationships? Think of some examples from your own life.
- In what ways is it possible for children and young people who have been separated from parents in the early years to compensate?

Further reading

For useful books to deepen understanding of attachment theory and the insights it offers into relationships, the following books are recommended:

Cassidy, J. & Shaver, P. R. (eds) (2008) *Handbook of Attachment: Theory, Research, and Clinical Applications*, 2nd edition, New York: Guilford Press.
Holmes, J. (1993) *John Bowlby and Attachment Theory*, London: Routledge.
Howe, D. (2005) *Child Abuse and Neglect: Attachment, Development and Intervention*, London: Palgrave Macmillan.
Prior, V. & Glaser, D. (2006) *Understanding Attachment and Attachment Disorders*, London: Jessica Kingsley.

The longitudinal ERA Study gives a unique perspective on the impact that early separation and neglect can have on children. For a summary, read: Rutter, M. *et al.* (2009) *Policy and Practice Implications from the ERA Study: Forty-Five Key Questions*, London: British Association for Adoption and Fostering. See also: Music, G. (2010) *Nurturing Natures: Attachment and Children's Emotional, Sociocultural and Brain Development*, London: Routledge, for an overview of the factors that influence children's development with especial focus on family and the social context.

Alternative perspectives on parenting can be found in: Golombok, S. (2000) *Parenting: What Really Counts?*, London: Routledge. See also: Goldberg, A. E. (2010) *Lesbian and Gay Parents and Their Children: Research on the Family Life Cycle*, Washington, DC: American Psychological Association and Pryor, J. & Rodgers, B. (2001) *Children in Changing Families: Life after Parental Separation*, Oxford: Basil Blackwell.

For a very insightful book on caring for troubled children, see: Hughes, D. A. (2006) *Building the Bonds of Attachment: Awakening Love in Deeply Troubled Children*, 2nd edition, Lanham, MD: Jason Aronson. See also: Archer, C. (1999) *Parenting the Child Who Hurts: First Steps – Tiddlers and Toddlers*, London: Jessica Kingsley, as well as Archer, C. (1999) *Parenting the Child Who Hurts: Next Steps – Tykes and Teens*, London: Jessica Kingsley, and Cairns, K. (2002) *Attachment, Trauma and Resilience. Therapeutic Caring for Children*, London: British Association for Adoption and Fostering.

Hayden, C. (2007) *Children in Trouble: The Role of Families, Schools and Communities*, Basingstoke: Palgrave, gives an evidence-based account of the multiple ways in which adults can improve or worsen the difficulties of children in trouble. Chapter 4 examines the role of families and considers the particular vulnerability of looked-after children. Hayden, C. & Gough, D. (2010) *Implementing Restorative Justice in Children's Residential Care*, Portland, OR: Polity Press, takes this further by examining the effectiveness of using restorative approaches for resolving conflicts among children and young people in residential care.

Websites and resources

The International Attachment Network, founded by Richard Bowlby, son of John Bowlby, provides information on attachment theory and runs bi-monthly workshops. The set of DVDs on attachment theory and practice is extremely useful:
http://www.attachmentnetwork.org/

See also the website of the British Association for Adoption and Fostering:
http://www.baaf.org.uk/

Chapter 4

Peer relationships in day care, nursery and school

Map of the chapter

This chapter examines the development of peer relationships in day care, nursery, school and the community. It explores how children relate to one another, and some of the difficulties that they encounter in their relationships with one another. It considers the controversies around the age at which pre-schoolers are ready to go to nursery or day care, and reports on research into the long-term effects of day care on children's emotional development. Different types of play activity are described, in particular, the value of imaginative play for emotional and social competence. This chapter considers the importance of friendships from pre-school through primary and secondary school, as well as the importance of sociometric status within the peer group. It also examines the issue of school bullying and strategies to overcome it. In the section on adolescence, the chapter considers the changing nature of relationships with same- and opposite-sex peers. It ends with a section on antisocial and prosocial behaviour in school and in the community.

The effects of day care on the under-twos

Clearly there are immense benefits to children when they interact with their peers and form friendships. Free early-years provision is now available in the UK for all 3- and 4-year-olds and currently round 97% of 4-year-olds and 87% of 3-year-olds are in some form of pre-school provision. But at what age before then are they ready to spend long periods of time away from their families? This is especially pertinent when mothers have to decide on the most appropriate age at which they can safely entrust their very young children to the care of others while they return to work after maternity leave.

From the attachment theory perspective, as indicated in Chapter 3, during the first year of life, children's attachments to primary caregivers are crucial. As a result, many mothers face a difficult decision if they need (or choose) to return to work while their children are very young. Many UK mothers – around 76% – return to work within 12 to 18 months of their child's birth. Some research indicates that there will be very few bad effects and a number of important benefits. For example, there is evidence that in deprived areas early intervention in the form of high-quality day care can compensate for risky family situations and help children develop social and emotional coping skills (Ramey *et al.*, 2000). However, other studies suggest that there are long-term risks of antisocial behaviour, emotional disturbance and mental health difficulties if children attend day care at a very early age. So it is important to be familiar with rigorous research studies on this topic. Here we focus on two major longitudinal studies, one in the USA (Belsky, 2006), the other in the UK (Sylva *et al.*, 2003).

A large project into the effects of routine, non-maternal childcare was carried out by Belsky and his team for the National Institute of Child Health and Human Development (NICHD) Early Child Care Research Network (ECCRN) (Belsky, 2006). This study followed 1,364 children from ten communities in the USA from birth through to the start of school at around the age of 5 years, and at regular points throughout the school years until 15 years of age. The aim of this research was to highlight the conditions under which early childcare experiences enhance or undermine children's cognitive, linguistic and socio-emotional development. One of the pressing social reasons for undertaking the research was the fact that a large percentage of mothers – as in the UK – were returning to work when their children were under the age of one year. So, more and more pre-schoolers were experiencing non-maternal care at younger and younger ages. The issue was especially influenced by scientific research findings on the importance of the child's relationship with the primary caregivers for later cognitive, social and emotional development. The concern was that there were risks associated with entering non-maternal day care during the very early years of life, including insecure attachment, and higher levels of aggression in the future at age 3–8 years and beyond. The study measured many aspects of children's development (social, emotional, intellectual, language development, behavioural problems and adjustment, and physical health). The children were given a range of measures at 6, 15, 24, 36 and 54 months and then again at regular points during their school years up to 15 years of age.

One aim of the study was to measure the security of children's attachment to primary care-givers. Belsky was aware that some critics of the Strange Situation Test as a test of attachment (e.g., Clarke-Stewart, 1989) had raised concerns that infants might be wrongly classified as insecure-avoidant (Type A) when in fact they were independent children, accustomed to separation from parents and reunions with them. So the research design included the measurement of children's responses to the Strange Situation Test as well as their responses to separation and reunion in more naturalistic contexts.

A second aim was to control for the effects of social class. It was possible that mothers who were obliged to return to work soon after the birth of their child might be from less advantaged backgrounds than mothers who could afford to stay at home to care for their baby. So Belsky and his team took account of socio-economic differences among the parents of the children in their sample. The backgrounds of the families were diverse, including low-income, single-parent and minority families. (But very few were extremely poor families enrolled in early intervention projects to compensate for disadvantage.)

Finally, the team made great efforts to gather evidence about the quality of the day care provision that the children experienced. Additionally, they took account of the time spent in day care and the age at which the children entered day care.

The major findings were as shown in Box 4.1.

Box 4.1

The effects of day care on child development (adapted from Belsky, 2006, 2010)

Childcare quality:

- Infants were more likely to develop insecure attachment to their mother when low-quality care coincided with low levels of maternal sensitivity.
- The more attentive and stimulating the childcare, the better the child's performance on cognitive and linguistic tasks at 15, 24 and 36 months. This finding also extended to tests of maths and reading achievement at 54 months, through to the third grade (8–9 years).
- The better the childcare, the fewer social and emotional behavioural difficulties and the greater the child's social competence at 24 and 36 months.
- Higher quality day care predicted more harmonious mother-child relationships across years 1–3 but from 54 months to first grade (6–7 years) this was only true if the children had experienced limited amounts of day care.

Childcare quantity:

- Evidence from this study indicated that time spent in care was related to attachment insecurity in interaction with other sources of risk. In other words, when mothers showed low levels of sensitivity to their infants at 6 and 15 months, and averaged more than 10 hours a week of day care, the infants were more likely to develop insecure attachment. This finding re-emerged when the Strange Situation Test was re-administered at 36 months.
- More time in care predicted elevated levels of externalizing problem behaviour as reported by caregivers at 24 months and 54 months. In other words, Clarke-Stewart's (1989) proposal that insecure children (as measured by the Strange Situation Test) were independent did not hold.
- Large amounts of time spent in day care throughout the infant, toddler and pre-school years predicted more aggression and disobedience in pre-

school and school, poorer relationships with teachers in elementary school and increased risk-taking with regard to alcohol, drugs and sexual behaviour by age 15 years.

Belsky (2006) concluded that early childcare from birth to 5 years is associated with developmental risks as well as benefits. The risks are that more hours spent in day care throughout the first 4–5 years of life are related to more risk of problem behaviour and less social competence at 54 months through to first grade. These risks persist through to adolescence. These effects are small but cumulatively they could have a large impact since so many small children are spending more and more time in day care during the pre-school years. The benefits are better cognitive, linguistic and academic achievement across the same developmental period.

Discussion questions

What are the implications for government policy of these findings? Should mothers of children under the age of 12 months return to work full time?

Sylva and her colleagues carried out two major studies in the *UK: Effective Provision of Pre-school Education* (EPPE) (Sylva *et al.*, 2003, 2004) and *Families, Children and Child Care* (Sylva *et al.*, 2009). EPPE tracked 3,000 UK children from 3 years of age and gathered retrospective data about their early years. The researchers found that children who had attended nursery had raised levels of aggression when they went to school at 5 years of age; this was still present at 7 years of age. But, they found, this disappeared by the time these children were 11 years of age. The EPPE project consistently found positive effects of high-quality pre-school provision on children's intellectual and social behavioural development up to the end of Key Stage 1 in primary school. The EPPE research indicates very importantly that the experience of *high-quality* pre-school provision is a critical way of overcoming social exclusion for disadvantaged children by giving them a better preparation for school life.

The *Families, Children and Child Care* Project (Sylva *et al.*, 2009) followed 1,000 babies from 3 months of age. The research team found no relationship between the amount of day care as a baby and behavioural problems at 3 years of age. However, Sylva added some cautionary warnings. There are no concerns about putting a child in nursery at 3 years of age. But between 2 and 3 years of age the outcomes are mixed, and below 18 months old there are some serious issues. After the age of 18 months, however, there seem to be advantages to being in day care. Children in day care have the opportunity to become more sociable with their peers and to learn valuable skills that will prepare them for school. The crucial aspect is that the childcare must be of a very high quality if it is to replicate a caring family environment. In confirmation, Leach *et al.* (2008) found that critical factors in day care included: the ratio of adults to children, the availability of caregivers who were attuned to the babies and empathic to their needs, and the provision of a rich, stimulating environment. Unfortunately, this study also found that, in comparison with non-maternal care from grandmothers, nannies and childminders, nurseries came out worse for babies under one year in terms of positive interactions and emotional sensitivity to the infants' needs.

The evidence from these studies provides crucial information on possible long-term effects of day care on children younger than a year but, since the findings differ in some respects, the situation remains that the researchers and childcare experts continue to disagree on this important matter. Belsky's concern was that the effect size of emotional and behavioural difficulties shown by children who had experienced day care at an early age was small, though statistically significant, but that difficulties persisted through to adolescence. Sylva, by contrast, argued that any negative effects 'wore off' by the time the children were 11 years of age. The two studies strongly advocate high-quality day care for the under-fives. They also support the recommendation that policies should support families in their search for good day care provision. There should be more support for parents who wish to work part time during the early years of their child's life.

Forming friendships in pre-school

From the age of 18 months, children demonstrate an increasing awareness of other children and respond by modifying their behaviour when in the presence of peers. There are immediate social and emotional benefits from interaction with peers. By the age of 2 or 3 years, most children are ready for nursery school or playgroup. The next sections explore the value of friendship and playful activity from pre-school right through to adolescence. From a very early age children are interested in their peers. Interactions between under-twos often consist of just looking at another child and maybe smiling or offering a toy. In toddler groups, these interactions are often quite short in duration. Adults can facilitate these interactions but much is initiated by the children themselves. So how do parents keep a good balance between ensuring that their young children feel safe and secure on the one hand and gain valuable opportunities to interact with same-age peers on the other?

Between 2 and 4 years old children's social skills develop as they interact with same-age others at nursery school or in day care where there are great opportunities for such activities as socio-dramatic play and rough-and-tumble play with peers. The development of friendships provides a vehicle for, and reflection of, increasing social understanding. Friendships and social networks play a critical role for emotional health and well-being. By the age of 2–3 years, children take delight in language games involving humorous rhymes, repetition of sounds and rhythms. By 3 years old they typically find the mislabelling of objects hilarious. They begin to appreciate jokes and riddles. Children use language extensively in their socio-dramatic play. By the age of 6, children begin to understand humour with multiple meanings.

The value of play

A great deal of time is spent throughout the pre-school and school years in play. Two- to four-year-olds demonstrate different kinds of activity when they are with their peers:

- *Solitary activity*: they play on their own even when in the company of other children;
- *Parallel play*: they play near one another with the same materials but do not interact much;
- *Cooperative play*: they interact together in complementary ways, e.g., getting toys from the cupboard and handing them to another child in order to initiate play.

Between 2 and 4 years of age, children become increasingly interested in cooperative activity, usually in groups of two or three children. Play has a number of very important functions for children: it helps to develop thinking and language; it helps children to deal with and understand emotions; it fosters the imagination; it provides a vehicle for interacting with other children. It can also have a healing function when children are upset or when they are experiencing difficult events in their lives (Cattanach, 1994). Children's capacity for play is greatly enhanced if they themselves feel secure (Stern, 2001). But, even in extreme circumstances, children play. For example, street children who are struggling to survive still find time to engage with others and with their environment through the medium of play. Where children are unhappy, play can be used as a form of therapy to enable them to explore issues of concern in a safe way (Fearn & Howard, 2012, in press). Sutton-Smith (2003) indicated the important role that play has for enabling children to act out and experience emotions without losing control. This can also serve a healing or therapeutic function and provide safe opportunities for regulating difficult emotions, such as anger, hurt and fear. Case Study 4.1 illustrates the value of play for children in extremely traumatic situations.

CASE STUDY 4.1

Play as a resource for children in adversity (adapted from Fearn & Howard, 2012, in press)

Fearn and Howard (ibid.) report findings from a case study (Abdunnur & Hartley, 2007) on the empowering effect of play for refugee children and young people in Beirut during the Israeli bombing in 2006. Abdunnur and a team of volunteers provided structured and dramatic play as an intervention to help alleviate the acute suffering that the children were experiencing. In particular, the volunteers introduced make-believe play through theatrical improvisation which the children later performed in front of audiences of 500 people from the community. Through this medium, the children were able to address the frightening circumstances in which they were living in the safe dramatic space where *they* could control the action and the outcomes. For the audience of friends and family, there was a brief respite from the horrors that surrounded them. The children's previous experiences of security from strong family and community networks provided the basis for this capacity to cope with trauma by harnessing the power of the imagination.

The authors conclude that imaginative play empowered the children to interact in a structured way with their chaotic environment, and to have an influence on it. This led to emotional regulation and helped to reduce the acute anxiety experienced by these children and young people. The authors argue strongly that there is a great need to provide children in difficult settings with the opportunity to play in order to build on their capacity for resilience.

Discussion question

Think of other situations in which children's resilience might be fostered through the experience of imaginative play.

Some researchers (e.g., Smith, 2010) propose that play evolves in a sequence from *functional* play (similar to practice play) to *constructive* play (making something, e.g., from Lego bricks), to *socio-dramatic* play (where children create scenarios and stories with characters) and finally to *games* with rules (e.g., the game of marbles). There are a number of different types of play: *locomotor* or physical activity play (covering *exercise* play, and *rough-and-tumble* play); *play with objects*; *fantasy* and *socio-dramatic* play; and *language* play (Box 4.2).

Box 4.2

Types of play (adapted from Smith *et al.*, 2011)

Physical activity play

Playful behaviour can be observed at a very early age. Babies engage in rhythmical movements as they kick their legs or wave their arms. These movements can be described as the precursors of play. During the pre-school years children engage in exuberant exercise play where they run around, jump and climb, either on their own or in the company of peers. Parents often facilitate this kind of play by tickling their pre-school children, chasing them and crawling around after them. By the primary school years, this physical activity evolves into rough-and-tumble play with peers.

Rough-and-tumble play

Play fighting, or rough-and-tumble play between peers, is common from 3 years of age through to adolescence and can involve wrestling, pushing, kicking and chasing. Although this kind of play can look aggressive, its playful nature is signalled by smiling and laughter. Children usually know the difference between real and play fighting. Play fights tend to be short in duration and the participants do not hurt one another. However, children who are rejected by their peers are more likely to mistake playful fighting for the real thing and retaliate in an aggressive manner.

Play with objects

From 2 years of age onwards, toddlers enjoy playing with objects, stacking and sorting blocks, doing simple jigsaws, arranging things by colour and size. Often this play is solitary but it forms the basis for later social play which requires shared attention to the objects concerned. A playful approach to objects fosters pretend play and the development of the imagination.

Fantasy and socio-dramatic play

The beginnings of fantasy play can be seen from about 12–15 months of age. Early pretend play is very literal and depends on actual objects, such as real cups and spoons. From 2 years of age onwards children are able to imagine scenarios and to make use of objects whatever they look like as props for the stories they are enacting. (For example, they can use any object to represent a toy weapon.) By 3 years of age, complex scripts have evolved with distinctive characters. Emotions are expressed that are appropriate to the events in the story. For 3–6-year-olds these scripts are often acted out with peers, each playing a different role or part in the script, such as: doctor/patient; mummy/daddy/child; king/queen/prince/princess. Language is important in these games.

Language play

Language play involves the playful use of sounds even before the child has mastered language. For example, the child will engage in repetitive play with syllables or with rhyming sounds, often in a rhythmic way.

Imaginary companions

Some children invent an imaginary companion who goes through all of the child's usual routines, such as going to bed, eating meals, getting ready to go out. These invisible friends typically have names, personalities and physical characteristics. Many creative children have imaginary friends onto whom they can project their dreams for the future as well as their fears and anxieties. The imaginary companion often has a key role to play in socio-dramatic play and can also be comforting when the child is lonely or distressed. Children will talk to the 'friend' about their problems, much as some children view their pets as close companions (Tatlow-Golden & Guerin, 2010). Research indicates that between 23% and 50% of children between 3 and 8 years of age have an imaginary companion. Asthana (2007) reports the work of Majors, an educational psychologist, who found the existence of imaginary companions in around 65% of children up to the age of 7 years. They were still present for 9% of 9-year-olds in her sample. The 'friends' were there when the children had difficulties and were also useful for taking the blame when things went wrong. Children are perfectly aware of the difference between these imaginary friends and real ones but the imaginary friends had a particular set of functions, essentially as one more way of helping the child to come to terms with the world around them. These invisible friends can do things that are impossible in everyday life and in this way can help the child to explore emotions and to practice new skills which can later be tested in the real world. The presence of the imaginary friend can also represent a step in the process of thinking abstractly since the companion is not literally there but lives in the world of the imagination. It is very important to enter into the child's imaginative world and not to dismiss the invisible friend as 'unreal' (Case Study 4.2).

CASE STUDY 4.2

Anna's imaginary friend, Pindy

When Anna, now a teacher of 6-year-olds, was a child she recalls that she had an imaginary friend called Pindy who was often present at meals or at bedtimes but who was never to be seen. Whenever Anna was worried about something she would discuss it with Pindy and whenever something went wrong in her life it was usually Pindy's fault. For example, when a toy was broken or some juice was spilt, Pindy would be there to take the blame. By the time Anna was 7 years of age, Pindy seemed just to go away but she lived on as a memory. Now that Anna works closely with young children she remembers how important it is to take such companions seriously in order to understand the world of the imagination.

Discussion questions

What function does an imaginary companion serve? Have you observed or experienced an imaginary companion? What were the benefits?

Sociometric status in the pre-school and at school

Even at pre-school, children can be categorized on the basis of their **sociometric status** types, as follows: *average*, *popular*, *controversial*, *rejected* or *neglected*, and these categorizations continue to be important during the school years. Interpersonal relationships continue to be very important as children move to primary school and it is important that they continue to experience school as a caring community. Significant adults continue to play a crucial role. Being supported by a caring adult can help children to see things from other points of view and to develop empathy for others. Caring relationships facilitate the growth of relationships based on trust and mutual respect. But increasingly, at this age, children are influenced by their social and emotional experiences with peers. Children who are emotionally skilled are more attractive as friends to their peers and so find it easier to form strong social support networks. For example, Petrides *et al.* (2006) found that children who rate highly on emotional intelligence are more likely to be perceived by their peers as having leadership qualities and being cooperative; they are less likely to be perceived as disruptive and aggressive. Children who are rejected or neglected by peers have a more stressful experience and are the focus of the following sections which cover relationship difficulties in childhood and adolescence. The sociometric categories are usually as follows:

- *Average* children have one or two mutual friends with whom they spend much of their time.
- *Popular* children are chosen by many of their peers as friends; they have good interpersonal skills; they are not especially aggressive nor are they withdrawn.
- *Controversial* children are aggressive but use this to gain status with their peers; they are both admired and feared by others.
- *Rejected* children tend to spend less time in cooperative play and social conversation and more time in arguing and fighting. They are more likely to interrupt games and try to disrupt other children's play. This behaviour tends to persist over time from pre-school onwards. Peer rejection in primary school is strongly related to psychopathology later on. It is important to help and support these children.
- *Neglected* children are low on sociability and tend not to be chosen as partners for activities or as friends in play. They spend more time in solitary play. They are quiet and can easily be overlooked. They too need help and support from adults.

In order to find out what are the factors that contribute to the competence of children and young people in making friends, a huge number of studies have been carried out on children's friendship choices. Pepler and Craig (1998) provide a useful review. These issues are explored in greater depth in the following sections which examine friends and enemies, ingroups and outgroups, as well as the widespread phenomenon of bullying and social exclusion during childhood and adolescence.

Ingroups and outgroups at school

Gender roles

Recent research indicates the crucial influence of the peer group on developing sex differences. Several studies have found that nursery school teachers tend to reward 'feminine' type behaviours (e.g., quiet, sedentary activities near an adult) in both boys and girls equally, yet this does not prevent boys engaging more than girls in noisy, rough-and-tumble play. This confirms the strong influence on children's constructs of their observations and experiences of playing and interacting with their peers. Throughout the pre-school years and into the school years, boys' and girls' peer groups differ. Boys' friendship groups tend to be bigger, more competitive and risk-taking while girls' groups are smaller and more intimate. Children not only selectively imitate same-sex models, but selectively observe and remember information that is relevant to or consistent with their own understanding of gender, or ignore and reject information that is not relevant or consistent with it. The child then focuses on a further understanding of their own gender identity through a grasp of the characteristics of their friendship group (Leman & Tenenbaum, 2011).

There are complex mechanisms at work here including:

- *Self-regulatory mechanisms* – children monitor their own behaviour with reference to what they consider to be appropriate for boys and girls;
- *Identification with a peer group* – children compare themselves with other same-sex peers;

● *Motivational mechanisms* – children are most likely to imitate behaviour which they think they can master and which will enhance their self esteem.

Children seem to practice future gender roles in their everyday activities with adults and peers, for example, as the next section indicates, in their expression of aggression. Even in pre-school, boys demonstrate more aggressive means of communication than girls and these differences seem to increase with age.

Interestingly, with regard to same-gender friendship preference, research by Zosuls *et al.* (2011) indicates that this reflects ingroup positivity rather than outgroup hostility. Whereas at nursery school, only around two-thirds of choice of playmate is same-sex, by the time that children go to primary school, sex segregation of children's groups is the norm. During the primary school years, there are distinct differences between the play of boys and girls. Boys are more likely to engage in competitive team games in large groups of mixed ages; the rules of the games become increasingly complex and are often the subject of intense debate and argument. Girls place more emphasis on small intimate groups or pairs, usually of same-age peers (Leman & Tenenbaum, 2011).

Schools have been a focus for work to foster tolerance among children. This can be assisted by a multi-ethnic curriculum approach that emphasizes the diversity of cultural beliefs and practices and gives them equal value, so bringing children of different ethnicities and nationalities together in common activities. For example, children are taught about relationships with others through the Social and Emotional Aspects of Learning (SEAL) curriculum. As indicated in Chapter 2, Humphrey *et al.* (2008) in their evaluation of SEAL in primary schools found that the programme acted as a bridge to behaviour within school but did not appear to transfer to home and community.

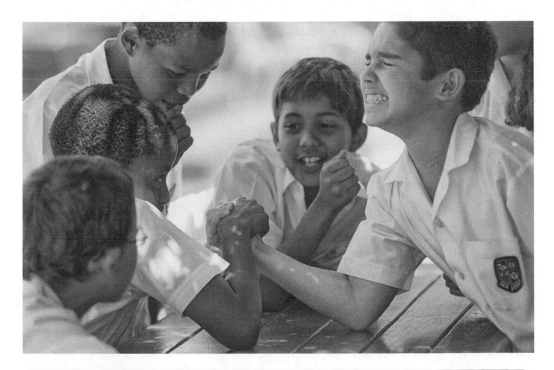

Justin Pumfrey/Getty images

Enemies

Children's peer relationships are extremely important to them and this topic has been widely researched. But a less researched area concerns childhood enemies. Card (2010), in a meta-analysis of 16 research studies on child and adolescent antipathetic relationships, found that the average prevalence rate was 35%. In other words, around one third of children and young people have at least one antipathetic relationship at any given time. Boys were slightly more likely than girls to have this kind of relationship but there were no significant differences by age. The research to date found no differences by ethnic group. Card was also interested to investigate whether there was a link with emotional difficulties and found that antipathetic relationships were associated with externalizing problems, such as aggression and disruptive behaviour, as well as with internalizing behaviours, such as depression and social withdrawal. They were also associated with victimization and rejection by peers and with having fewer friends. Another interesting finding was that a substantial number of 'enemies' were former friends whose relationship had been undermined by some violation, such as breaking trust or telling an intimate secret. A proportion of children continue to need additional support and in some schools there are Nurture Groups to help children with social, emotional and behavioural difficulties (see Chapter 2).

CASE STUDY 4.3

Becky's letter to a teen magazine

My friend has a boyfriend who she really likes but she keeps talking about him which is making me jealous because I never get boyfriends. I don't know what to do about how I feel. Becky, 14

Discussion question

How would you answer Becky's letter?

Aldrich *et al.* (2011) used a narrative method to elicit children's perceptions of jealousy in relationships. They found interesting age differences: 5–6-year-olds tended to focus on the basic emotion of anger, whereas 7–8-year-olds spoke of a variety of emotions, including jealousy, unhappiness, anger, sadness and annoyance. These findings suggest that the child's conception of jealousy begins with a negative feeling and increasingly develops in complexity as the child understands additional relevant information. The older children in this study were much more able to identify a rival and to take the perspective of others.

Ethnic preference

Strong feelings of positivity and negativity are not only confined to individual relationships. They also apply to whole groups. In this context, it is important to consider the nature of attitudes held by children and young people towards ingroups and outgroups in their society (Oppenheimer & Barrett, 2011). Of relevance here is the young person's growing awareness of their own *ethnic identity* – that is, their awareness of their membership of a particular national or social group. Earlier research into ethnic preference used black and white dolls or photographs to elicit children's choices and attributions. It was found that children of 4 years and over tended to choose the doll or photograph of someone from their own ethnic group. On the basis of this methodology, Aboud (1988) concluded that dissimilar people were disliked and proposed that children were prone to racial prejudice from around 6 years of age. More recent research (Barrett, 2007; Barrett *et al.*, 2003; Oppenheimer & Barrett, 2011) has challenged such interpretations on the grounds that the measurement of positive choices towards the ingroup does not necessarily imply negative attitudes towards the outgroup. For example, Takriti *et al.* (2000), in a study of Muslim and Christian children aged from 5 to 11 years, found a shift away from assigning mainly positive attributes to the ingroup and mainly negative attributes to the outgroup at 5 years of age, to assigning both positive and negative attributes to both ingroup and outgroup by 11 years of age.

Barrett (2007) designed a more complex measure, the Strength of Identification Scale (SoIS), to elicit the views of children and young people towards their own national state and towards different ethnic, racial or religious groups. In the SoIS, participants are asked to assign different positive and negative qualities to people of different countries, including their own country or national group, the 'traditional enemy' outgroup, and other more neutral outgroups. Using the SoIS, in a study of 594 6-year-olds from five culturally diverse nations – Azerbaijan, the UK, Georgia, Russia and Ukraine – Bennett *et al.* (2004) found, as predicted, that the children showed preference for people who shared their own nationalities. However, in very few cases was there negative evaluation of the outgroups. In fact, in some instances there was outgroup popularity (e.g., in the UK about French and Spanish outgroups, and in Georgia and Ukraine about Armenian and Russian outgroups). Typically, attitudes towards outgroups were neutral. In other words, there was no evidence that commitment to one's own national identity resulted in prejudice against the outgroup. The exception was where that outgroup presented a threat to a nation. For example, Azeri children expressed negative views about Russians, an understandable finding since Russia had supported the Armenians when they occupied Azeri territory in 1992.

These studies indicate how essential it is to take account of the socio-historical context in which children are growing up in order to gauge the complexity of their attitudes towards ingroups and outgroups. As Barrett and Oppenheimer (2011) indicate, on the basis of a range of studies, there is considerable variation in the attitudes that children express towards different national groups throughout middle childhood. Sometimes with age they become more negative, sometimes more positive, sometimes they change from positive to negative, or from negative to positive. Sometimes they remain stable. These patterns seem to be related to a number of factors, including the perceived characteristics of the outgroup, the national context within which the child is growing up, and the child's own specific geographical, ethnic and linguistic position within that national context.

In contemporary society, where there are large migrations of people from other cultures, there are important implications for the role of schools in multi-ethnic communities in teaching tolerance and cooperation, and in emphasizing the value of diversity in deepening understanding of cultures other than one's own. In the next section, the focus is on young people's perspectives on the rights of refugee children.

Young people's perceptions of the rights of asylum-seeking children

Some research indicates that mainstream adolescents and children often hold prejudiced views of marginalized and disadvantaged peers, for example, towards sexual minority youth (Rivers, 2011), ethnic minority youth (Killen & Stangor, 2001) and disabled youth (Norwich & Kelly, 2004). They may also hold negative views towards refugees in the light of differences in cultural practices and religion. Ruck *et al.* (2007) investigated the views of 60 adolescents (30 were in the early to middle adolescence age group and 30 were in late adolescence) about the rights of asylum-seeking children. They used vignettes, each involving a 12-year-old refugee matched to the participant's gender. Two of the vignettes described a situation where the asylum-seeker child wished to exercise a self-determination right (such as choosing where to live, or refusing to carry an ID card) in the context of conflict with government or authority practices; the other two vignettes described a situation where the 12-year-old refugee wanted to have a nurturance right upheld (such as being provided with money, food and clothing) that was in conflict with the authorities. They found that in each of the age groups the participants favoured the asylum-seeker children's nurturance rights over their self-determination rights. They used distinct forms of reasoning for the two categories of rights. With regard to nurturance rights, they used moral-based reasoning, including reference to fairness and empathy. With regard to self-determination rights, they used social conventional reasoning (e.g., maintaining group functioning) and psychological reasoning (e.g., personal choice). In other words, in this study, providing care and protection was viewed more as a matter for moral concern than providing opportunities for independent decision-making or autonomy. There were strong gender differences too. Older females were significantly more likely to endorse children's self-determination rights than males. This finding was explained as possibly being due to the fact that young women are more likely to have encountered unfair treatment than young men and so have greater sensitivity to unfair treatment surrounding civil liberties and self-determination rights. This research is important in the light of fostering better understanding of intergroup relations and in the promotion of human rights as countries become increasingly multi-ethnic.

Bullying and social exclusion

Unfortunately, children's relationships do not always go smoothly. Boys of all ages are more likely to experience physical bullying, while girls are more likely to experience indirect forms, such as being left out or ignored, having false rumours spread, or being given dirty looks. Friendship is an important protective factor, but so too is the active intervention of bystanders, often those with high empathy for the distress of others as well as high status among the peer group. There are very damaging outcomes for children who are bullied by their peers, especially when it is long term (Cowie & Jennifer, 2008). The bullied child's self-esteem is likely to suffer and this may lead to mental health difficulties. Children who bully are also at risk. There is evidence that they are more likely as adults to be involved in criminal activity and domestic violence (Farrington, 1995; Farrington & Baldry, 2010). Bullying takes a number of forms:

- *Psychological bullying:* involves spreading malicious rumours about another person, excluding a person from the group, disclosing someone's secrets;
- *Physical bullying:* includes such behaviours as hitting, pushing, punching or kicking;
- *Cyberbullying:* refers to a form of covert psychological bullying using electronic devices, such as e-mail, mobile phones, text messages, video clips, instant messaging, photos and personal websites in order to engage in repeated hostile behaviour intended to harm a person.

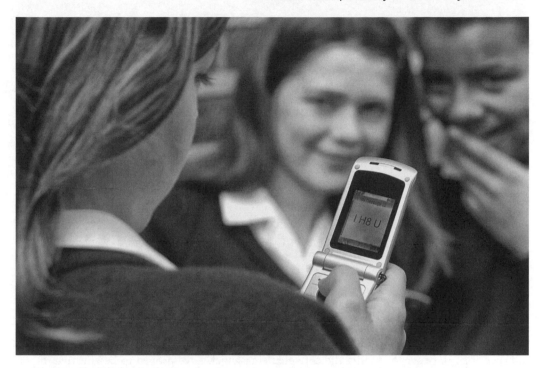

Chris Whitehead/Getty images

Box 4.3

Types of bully (adapted from Cowie & Jennifer, 2008: 55)

Bullies can be classified into a number of categories, as follows:

Aggressive bullies: These are most likely to be the ringleader bullies. Typically, they are low in empathy for others' suffering. They are manipulative, impulsive, assertive, strong and easily provoked; they take the lead in initiating the aggression; they often seek out other bullies to form a coterie of followers who join in with their aggressive behaviour and support it.

Anxious bullies/assistants to the bully: In contrast to the leadership qualities of the aggressive bully, they are followers, possibly to compensate for their own feelings of insecurity. They often appear desperate for approval from the aggressive bullies.

Reinforcers of the bully: Like the assistants to the bully, the reinforcers are part of the coterie of followers. Their role is to encourage the ringleader bully by, for example, laughing, actively watching the episode, providing an audience for the ringleader's aggressive behaviour.

Bully-victims: Bully-victims are the most emotionally disturbed since they are aggressive towards their peers but are also the target of their peers' aggression.

Discussion question

Try to link these different types of bully to secure and insecure attachment types.

Intervening to prevent and reduce bullying

International evaluation studies (Baldry & Farrington, 2007; Smith *et al.*, 2004a; Ttofi & Farrington, 2009) have systematically reviewed the successes and failures of anti-bullying interventions in order to identify the core elements which have proved to be effective. It is a common-sense view that the best approach to the prevention of bullying is to mete out punishment to the bullies. However, research indicates that this approach can be counter-productive. Skiba *et al.* (2008), in their report to the American Psychological Association Zero Tolerance Task Force, concluded that punitive, zero-tolerance policies actually failed to make school environments safer. They also observed that zero-tolerance policies can be construed as racist in the local community. Black parents/caregivers, in this study, became very critical of schools if they perceived that punitive zero-tolerance disciplinary methods and sanctions posed a threat to the rights of certain children to be educated, particularly when, as often happens, certain ethnic groups appeared to be targeted. Skiba and colleagues concluded that far more emphasis needs to be placed on the host of existing strategies that promote school safety and prevent bullying and violence. Zero-tolerance strategies should only be used in the most extreme and severe cases of bullying and even then used with great thought for the needs and rights of all the individuals involved, including the bullies. Based on this evidence it would seem that authoritarian, punitive use of sanctions is not a good approach.

In their Campbell Collaborative Report, Ttofi and Farrington (2009) reviewed 89 evaluations of anti-bullying programmes. They found that the most important elements in reducing bullying included training and meetings with parents as well as clear sanctions, such as serious talks with bullies, sending them to the head teacher, making them stay close to the teacher during break time, and depriving them of privileges. Similarly, Smith *et al.* (2004a) found that when schools promoted an emphasis on positive relationships and created an ethos of care and responsibility, the need for strict sanctions declined. When sanctions *were* applied, the perpetrators were more likely to perceive them as fair and meaningful. The reason for this was that the students had been included in the process of creating the school rules and had been made aware that negative behaviour, such as bullying, had consequences. So the sanctions were not perceived as unreasonably punitive.

So, the evidence seems to point to the effectiveness of sanctions that are perceived by children and young people as fair and reasonable rather than harsh punishment. Sanctions also need to be consistently applied and their design needs to be part of a consultation process in which many members of the school and its community have played a part. Sanctions need to be viewed in the wider context of the whole school and its values.

The Olweus Bullying Prevention Program

An example of the successful implementation of the whole-school approach can be seen in the Olweus Bullying Prevention Program (Olweus, 1993), described in Box 4.4.

Box 4.4

The Olweus Bullying Prevention Program (adapted from Olweus, 1993) http://www.olweus.org/public/bullying_prevention_program.page

The Olweus Bullying Prevention Program operates at three levels of intervention:

School-wide interventions
- Administration of the Olweus Bully/Victim Questionnaire about bullying (answered anonymously by the students)
- Formation of a Bullying Prevention Coordinating Committee
- Staff training
- Development of school-wide rules against bullying
- Development of a coordinated system of supervision during break time

Classroom-level interventions
- Regular classroom meetings about bullying and peer relations
- Class-parent meetings

Individual-level interventions
- Individual meetings with children who bully
- Individual meetings with children who are targets of bullying
- Meetings with parents of children involved

A key aspect of the Olweus Bullying Prevention Program is the development of a Bullying Prevention Coordinating Committee which contains representatives of school staff, students, parents and the coordinator of the program. Teachers take part in initial training and hold regular classroom meetings to monitor the development of the intervention.

Olweus (ibid.) argues that an authoritative rather than authoritarian adult-child interaction, involving an emotionally warm climate and clear rules, lies at the heart of an effective anti-bullying approach. This approach must by its nature be absorbed by parents and caregivers in the community, particularly as they are often the first adults to notice when their child is distressed. The

---

school needs to work hard to overcome any potential barriers, for example, when the origins of the aggressive behaviour lie in the family itself. Therefore, it is essential for the professionals in the school setting to communicate with the parents/caregivers as partners in educating children to relate to one another in respectful, caring and supportive ways. Schools, parents/caregivers and the community are in a much stronger position to counteract bullying if they are able to work constructively together in a responsible way for the best interests of the children in their care.

Discussion question

Why is it so important to consult with members of the whole-school community when planning anti-bullying interventions?

Helping the victims

Some children are able to deal with bullying experiences by using their own inner resources to cope with the distress of being bullied; others try out a range of strategies in order to escape the bullying. These young people provide useful information about how to help bullied peers. In one longitudinal study carried out in 35 UK schools over a period of two years (Cowie, 2002; Smith *et al.*, 2004a), the researchers asked the children how they coped with being bullied. They found that 'escaped victims' (those who were no longer being bullied after a period of two years) did not differ substantially from non-victims in terms of their personal characteristics or the type of bullying that they experienced. However, what did differentiate them was their resilience in developing effective coping strategies. The pupils who had escaped from being bullied reported a number of effective strategies, such as telling someone, actively trying to make new friends and even befriending the bully – strategies which the 'continuing victims' (those who had been bullied for more than two years) were less likely to display. The continuing victims had a significantly worse attendance rate at school in this study – a strategy that probably only served to isolate them further from their peers. They were also more likely to blame themselves. The young people who escaped had developed resilience in the face of adversity.

Box 4.5

Effective coping strategies for victims (adapted from Cowie, 2002)

Telling someone: By reporting a bullying incident to someone, you are taking the first step towards dealing with the problem and trying to find a solution. This is not a sign of weakness, though domineering peers may say that it is. It is important for schools to promote a climate in which it is safe to talk about issues that worry you.

Having a friend: Having at least one good friend at school is a fundamental resource for those having problems with bullying. It can also be a real strategy when the victimized pupil starts a process of getting new friends in order to cope with the bullying.

Nonchalance: Making out that you don't care and it doesn't affect you can be an effective strategy, especially if you have an inner sense that bullying is unjust and wrong. This is quite different from passively accepting the situation. Nonchalance is not just ignoring the fact but having a positive attitude not to let it get you down.

Get involved in your school's peer support scheme: These schemes take a number of forms but they are all designed to take an active stance against bullying. Often children who have been helped by peer supporters want to return the benefit in some way by helping others in distress. One immediate outcome is that you gain a helpful circle of friends.

Discussion questions

Thinking back to your school days, how effective do you think that these strategies would have been? Can you think of others that would be equally effective?

Friendships in adolescence

Friendship continues to be of intense importance during adolescence. As adolescents become independent from their parents, they spend more time with peers and turn to peers rather than adults for social support. During the primary-school years children's friendships are usually with people of the same sex. By early adolescence, both boys and girls continue to participate in groups, often of same-sex peers. Much of their energy is focused on same-sex relationships with large amounts of time spent in talking, chatting online, engaging in shared activities and interests.

At the same time, from around 11–13 years of age, both boys and girls express strong anxiety about their friendships, with a great deal of worry about the possibility of being rejected by peers. This anxiety seems to peak at 14–15 years of age and decrease from 16 years of age onwards. The pressure to conform to the opinions and attitudes of the peer group is strong but is also counterbalanced in many young people by an equally strong need to form their own independent views (Steinberg & Monahan, 2007).

CASE STUDY 4.3

Letter to the problem page of a teen magazine

All my friends are so pretty and popular. It makes me feel really low on confidence. They get all the guys and always look great and I don't. What should I do? Anon, aged 13

Discussion question

How would you answer this letter?

By adolescence, and with the onset of puberty, young people are increasingly interested in forming romantic/sexual relationships. In the early stages of adolescence, these partnerships are quite short-lived but the duration of intimate partnerships increases steadily with age. Although birth control methods are available to adolescents, there is quite wide variation in the extent to which they are actually used, with a proportion of young people regularly engaging in risky behaviour, such as unprotected sex and multiple partners (see Chapter 7).

Broadly, the development of romantic heterosexual partner relationships goes through the following stages (Brown, 1999):

- *Initiation phase*: awakening of interest in the opposite sex; but dating is very much bound up with existing friendships with same-sex peers who are frequently consulted and involved in the dating process; there can be conflicts here too if the best friend feels left out by the new romantic partner;
- *Status phase*: romantic relationships mainly seen in the context of status with same-sex peers, the aim being to achieve a high-status romantic partner;
- *Affection phase*: here there is a shift of focus onto the romantic relationship itself and the peer group has less influence; there is growing commitment to the relationship, often with increased sexual activity;
- *Bonding phase*: as adolescents get older, the romantic relationship is more likely to be seen as a long-term commitment.

Young people use romantic/sexual relationships as safe havens, similar to, but not identical to, the secure base that they experienced as infants. Sexual partners can become attachment figures to whom they can transfer their attachment needs for intimacy and emotional support (Hazan & Zeifman, 1994). A proportion of young people (around 5–7%) will come out as gay or lesbian at some point during adolescence. While awareness of sexual orientation emerges from around the age of 10 years, 'coming out' openly as gay or lesbian is often a very difficult process for young people since they may anticipate negative reactions from friends and family (Rivers & Gordon, 2010). Young lesbian and gay people also face the challenge of deciding whether it is safe to disclose their sexual orientation to a same-sex friend. Reactions to 'coming out' are varied and are often strongly influenced by the attitudes of the wider society or the local community in which the family of the young person lives. The responses of the peer group are also critical (Willoughby *et al.*, 2006).

There is some evidence that those who were securely attached as infants generally have greater likelihood of having positive experiences of intimacy in their romantic/sexual relationships, whereas those who were classified as insecure/ambivalent (Type C) are more likely to have turbulent relationships (Davila *et al.*, 2004; Mayseless & Scharf, 2007).

Pro- and antisocial behaviour in adolescence

The influence of the peer group is particularly strong during mid-adolescence for those engaged in antisocial behaviour, a loosely defined term for a range of activities from non-criminal to criminal that varies according to cultural tolerance and levels of what the public deems to be acceptable (Rogers, 2010). There seems to be a large discrepancy between public perception of antisocial behaviour on the part of youth and official records, with the UK public and the media consistently overestimating the extent of youth involvement in crime. Furthermore, the press reports frequently imply that violent crime is endemic within ethnic minority communities in a way that ignores other contributory factors, such as discrimination, disadvantage and inequality. Youth is often labelled negatively in the media with such sensationalist headlines as 'out-of-control gangs', 'Britain's growing knife menace' and 'lawless teens' (Sveinson, 2008: 14).

According to a report based on the British Crime Survey and the Police Recorded Crime (Kershaw *et al.*, 2008), adults' most frequently cited example of antisocial behaviour was 'teenagers hanging around in the streets' (31%). In one study that investigated the issue from the young person's perspective (Rogers, 2010: 200), however, there was resentment that boys got into trouble just for hanging about 'even if we're not up to anything, because we look dodgy', though they did admit that sometimes they were noisy and engaged in nuisance behaviour.

Box 4.6

Prejudiced perspectives on youth crime

In a report funded by the Runnymede Trust, Sveinson (2008) carried out a systematic analysis of articles in the national press over a period of two months. The report argues that violent crime is portrayed as endemic within minority ethnic communities but, at the same time, unrelated to the structure of British society. Media reports of crime, especially violent teenage crime, habitually use the concept of 'culture' to explain gang, gun and knife violence. The outcome is that too often the press connects criminal 'cultures' to specific ethnic communities with the false implication that most members of these communities are violent. In essence, Sveinson argues that England is conceived as twofold: an England of law-abiding Us and an England of criminal and violent Others.

Discussion question

To what extent do you agree with Sveinson's interpretation of media coverage of youth crime?

Deviant subcultures in adolescence

Membership of deviant groups in adolescence can be a serious problem both for the individuals involved and for their community. There is evidence for schoolyard 'corner' societies displaying antisocial behaviour within school. It is common in adolescence for young people to engage in some risky behaviour which, in a proportion of cases, can be described as antisocial behaviour, including substance abuse, excessive drinking, shoplifting, experimenting with drugs. Young people will often seek out the company of similar peers who in turn reinforce the risky behaviour and give it status.

In order to counteract such antisocial behaviour, schools must develop behaviour policies that indicate the following:

- Shared vision throughout the school about what is and is not acceptable behaviour;
- Students have some control over what happens to them at school;
- Discipline policies are perceived to be fair, firm and consistent;
- Discipline policies are not based on harsh punitive approaches;
- The school regularly rewards students for positive behaviour.

Membership of a gang goes beyond the minor antisocial behaviour that we have described above. The emphasis instead tends to be on the relationship between 'street' or 'ethnic' gangs and their immediate community. Membership is linked to aggressiveness and gangs are characterized by:

- Prohibited behaviour;
- Defiance of authority figures, such as teachers, police, social workers;
- Leadership in a structured group;
- Frequent association among gang members;
- Antagonism towards some outside reference group(s), such as other gangs;
- Often some territorial identification, for example, within certain boundaries in a particular neighbourhood.

Although previously gang membership was largely male, there is evidence more recently for an increase of girls' involvement in gangs. Some girls find gang members attractive and girls who are sexually mature early may also gravitate towards antisocial groups. Gangs often arouse fear in other young people and in adults. This power to intimidate can be very rewarding to young people whose identity and status is bound up with dominance and aggression. Antagonism to society at large can be especially rewarding to gang members and helps to strengthen the relationships within the gang.

As Wood and Alleyne (2010) propose, the ways in which the media report crime can often give a distorted impression of the ethnic composition of gangs. Although a gang can contain both black and white youth, young black criminality is more often associated with 'gang membership', so leading to an illogical assumption that certain ethnic groups are responsible for a disproportionate amount of crime.

Prosocial action during adolescence

There is widespread public awareness of antisocial behaviour during adolescence and frequently expressed views that young people are cynical or disengaged from society. What is often less emphasized is the prevalence of prosocial behaviour during this time. Cremin *et al.* (2011) reviewed existing studies of young people and their civic action; they also gathered data from a range of voluntary organizations working with young people from disadvantaged communities. They found that many young people in disadvantaged circumstances were civically engaged in their communities and, as a result, were making important contributions to their families and communities. The researchers defined civic action as 'an active concern for the common good' that ranged from concerned interest and informal volunteering (e.g., babysitting) through to politicized direct action. Here are two examples, derived from focus groups with young people (ibid.: 8), which indicate the perceived benefits of engaging in civic action, both for the giver and the receiver:

> You know, for me it's becoming a canoeing instructor, that was it for me, and I finally found something I was good at and I no longer cared about that group of friends that had been insulting me for five years, or whatever. Because actually I found something I was good at, where I fitted in and people would say, 'Actually, do you know what, well done.'
>
> (Adolescent girl)

> We're the ones that are in care, and it's like we're the ones that people are gonna turn to if they've got a problem . . . It's like . . . It's like we're, I don't know, listeners for them.
>
> (Looked-after young man)

The researchers identified the following intrinsic and extrinsic benefits reported by these young people:

- *Education and employment opportunities* though accreditation, learning basic skills, networking, obtaining references, learning how to deal with the system;
- *Developing soft skills* including confidence, teamwork, self-discipline, developing maturity and tolerance;
- *Being valued* through having a voice and having a sense of achievement;
- *Making a difference* to their own lives and communities;
- *Greater social cohesion* through meeting new people and challenging prior conceptions.

(Cremin *et al.*, 2011: 11)

Chapter summary

This chapter examined the course of the development of peer relationships among children and young people, and charted their progress in day care, school and the community. It began by considering the value and risks of day care at different ages during the early years. Then it charted friendship in the pre-school years, including the value of cooperative and imaginative play in enhancing social and emotional competence. It identified some of the difficulties in peer relationships experienced by children and young people, including having enemies and being bullied. Gender issues were explored in the context of adolescent same- and opposite-sex relationships. The chapter ended by discussing pro- and antisocial behaviour in adolescence.

Discussion points

- At what age can pre-schoolers be left safely in day care?
- Is adolescence automatically a time of storm and stress?
- What are the most effective methods for counteracting school bullying?

Further reading

Dunn, J. (2004) *Children's Friendships: The Beginnings of Intimacy*, Oxford: Basil Blackwell, is an excellent account of the significance of children's early friendships for their emotional health and well-being. See also: Bagwell, C. L. & Schmidt, M. E. (2011) *Friendships in Childhood and Adolescence*, New York: Guilford Press.

Branch, C. (ed.) (1999) *Adolescent Gangs: Old Issues, New Approaches*, New York: Taylor & Francis, approaches the issue of adolescent gangs from a range of disciplinary perspectives and provides useful insights into community-based interventions as well as mental health-based interventions.

Smith, P. K. (2010) *Children and Play*, Oxford: Wiley-Blackwell, is a good source of recent research and thinking on play. Singer, D. G. & Singer, J. L. (2005) *Imagination and Play in the Electronic Age*, Cambridge, MA: Harvard University Press, covers a variety of important topics including war play and computer games.

Rivers, I. & Gordon, K. (2010) '"Coming out", context, and reason: first disclosure of sexual orientation and its consequences', *Psychology and Sexuality*, 1(1): 21–33, is an up-to-date review of the experiences of young people when they come out to family and friends.

Rogers, R. A. (2010) 'Soft benefits for hard nuts: the impact of community-building interventions on "anti-social" youth', *Pastoral Care in Education*, 28(3): 195–204, is a readable account of ways in which collective action can help to reduce antisocial behaviour on the part of youth.

Ross, D. M. (2003) *Childhood Bullying, Teasing and Violence: What School Personnel, Other Professionals and Parents Can Do*, Alexandria, VA: American Counseling Association, gives comprehensive advice, grounded in research findings, on how to address the issue of school bullying. Further insights can be found in: Finkelhor, D. (2007) *Childhood Victimization: Violence, Crime, and Abuse in the Lives of Young People*, Oxford: Oxford University Press.

For a comprehensive account of restorative practices in schools and in residential care, see: Hopkins, B. (2011) *Just Care: Restorative Justice Approaches to Working with Children in Public Care*, London: Jessica Kingsley.

To follow up recent research on children's ethnic preferences, see the Special Issue on national identity and ingroup/outgroup attitudes in children edited by Oppenheimer, L. & Barrett, M. (2011) 'National identity and in-group/out-group attitudes in children: the role of sociohistorical settings. An introduction to the special issue', *European Journal of Developmental Psychology*, 8(1): 1–4.

Clark, M. M. & Tucker, S. (eds) (2010) *Early Childhoods in a Changing World*, Stoke-on-Trent: Trentham Books, examines the effects on young children's lives of changes in family circumstances, such as poverty, social isolation and trauma. This book contains fascinating case studies and personal narratives.

See: Howe, C. (2010) *Peer Groups and Children's Development*, Chichester: Wiley/Blackwell, for a scholarly account of the influence of the peer group on the social and cognitive development of children and young people.

Websites and resources

Takeover Day is a nationwide initiative organized by the Children's Commissioner to involve children and young people in decision-making in their schools and communities:
www.childrenscommissioner.gov.uk/takeover_day

ENVISION is an organization that challenges negative stereotypes about young people by helping them to design their own local community projects:
www.envision.org.uk

Plings provides opportunities for young people from 13 to 19 years of age to realize diverse ambitions, unexpected interests and to share lifestyle-changing experiences. Its aim is to develop young people's potential by inspiring them to make changes:
www.plings.net

For a range of useful coping strategies for bullied children, visit the ChildLine website:
http://www.childline.org.uk/explore/bullying/pages/bullying.aspx

Belinda Hopkins's website Transforming Conflict provides a range of useful resources on anti-bullying methods and restorative practices. These include information on the DVD *Introducing Restorative Justice: A Positive Approach in Schools*:
http://www.transformingconflict.org/resources.html

Chapter 5

Language and communication

Map of the chapter

This chapter examines some major theories of language development. It considers the impact of infant-directed speech (IDS) and child-directed speech (CDS) on the child's language development. Then it considers language in its cultural context, including the role of adults and peers in guiding children's communication skills. It highlights the importance of narrative and storytelling in developing children's mind-mindedness, and the importance of this in facilitating the transition from oracy to literacy. The intersubjectivity involved in mind-mindedness remains extremely important in developing pre-reading and pre-writing skills, and continues to have an impact as children progress through primary and secondary school. The chapter concludes by examining some literacy programmes in schools as well as methods, including collective argumentation, that facilitate the development of thinking and critical skills through collaborative discussion.

Introduction

Language competence is crucial for emotional well-being, social functioning and thinking capacity across the lifespan and in all cultures. As Snow (2009) indicates, language is both a *predictor* variable in infancy and an *outcome* variable in later childhood and in the mature years. As with other aspects of development, there is quite wide variation in the ages at which children reach specific milestones in language development, though the sequences tend to be similar. Most babies are competent communicators long before the emergence of the first words. Children appear to be programmed to learn language but the adults and children in the child's immediate environment play a huge part in facilitating language development.

By the end of the first year, most children can attract the attention of others, communicate a range of emotions, make clear their requests and make comments using non-verbal strategies. There are four key areas of language that the child must master:

1 *Phonology* refers to the system that governs the particular sounds (or phonemes) used in the language of a child's community in order to convey meaning. For example, an English speaker treats the sounds 'l' and 'r' as two separate phonemes; to a Japanese speaker they are one. Scottish people use the speech sound 'ch' (as in 'loch'). These phonemes are combined into syllables, morphemes (the smallest meaningful linguistic unit) and words.

2 *Semantics* refers to the meanings encoded in language. Phonemes are in themselves meaningless but they are combined to form morphemes, the smallest meaningful units of language. These may be whole words ('cat' in English, 'chat' in French) or grammatical markers, such as '-ed' at the end of a verb to make the past tense. The child learns that morphemes, words and longer utterances refer to events, people, objects, relationships, in short, that they convey meaning.

3 *Syntax* refers to the form and order in which words are combined to make grammatical sentences. The child progresses, for example, from saying 'Ben cup' to saying 'Ben wants that red cup.' The rules that govern such sequences are known as *syntax*. The term *grammar* refers to the study of the rules that determine sequences of morphemes and words in any language. These grammatical rules determine how words and morphemes in a language can be combined and sequenced to produce meaningful sentences.

4 *Pragmatics* is knowledge about how language is used in different contexts. The young child must learn to adapt her language to the situation in which she finds herself. A toddler may shout out loudly in the restaurant, 'That man's got no hair!' The sentence shows understanding of phonology, syntax and semantics, but lacks sensitivity to others' feelings.

There are several theories of language development based on a large body of experimental and observation data. From one broad perspective, the focus is on the internal processes in the child's mind; another perspective emphasizes the social and cultural contexts within which the child learns language; still further perspectives emphasize intersubjectivity between child and adult. For a comprehensive critical overview, see Saxton (2010).

Chomsky's (1965, 1986) theory proposed that all languages have a general form which he termed **universal grammar**. By this he meant that humans possess an innate, universal predisposition to language. To Chomsky, the environmental input that children receive was simply not enough to explain the extraordinary rapidity with which they acquire language. The inputs from adults must, he argued, be triggering an existing universal grammar. In the light of his proposition that languages have universal properties, including phonological aspects (consonants, vowels and syllables) and a grammatical structure, Chomsky argued that humans have an innate **language acquisition device (LAD)** without which language could not develop. According to Chomsky's theory, all languages have deep structures (the underlying meaning) and surface structures (the ordering of words in a sentence) which are linked through the rules of transformation, which make the connection between sound and meaning in any given language. Since the LAD can acquire any language, the child is involved in a creative process of generating language by applying transformational rules. Even their early utterances, for example, 'teddy chair' (meaning 'teddy's chair') or 'chair broken' (meaning 'the chair is broken'), can be classified as grammatical since they appear to demonstrate the systematic use of rules.

More recently, Pinker (1994, 2007) points to confirmatory evidence that in many communities in the world parents do not engage in the child-directed speech so prominent in the West, yet their children learn to speak. This viewpoint is vehemently contested by Saxton (2010: 102) and we return to the issue later in this chapter. However, further evidence that confirms Chomsky's theory comes from studies of **pidgin languages** which typically do not have consistent word order, tenses or any structures more complex than simple clauses. For example, Bickerton (1990) investigated pidgin language in Hawaii, developed by labourers who were imported from a wide range of countries to work in the plantations and who did not share a common language. In order to communicate, they spontaneously developed pidgin, a mixture of all the languages that they heard in their daily life. However, the children of these labourers were born in Hawaii and, out of the pidgin that they heard the adults speak, they developed their own language, now called Hawaiian Creole, which *is* grammatical, has standardized word orders, markers for present, future and past tenses, and subordinate clauses. In different parts of the world, **Creole languages**, which evolve out of unrelated language mixtures such as pidgin, provide support for the concept of a universal grammar that underlies all languages.

Similar confirmation came from research into sign language (Morford & Kegl, 2000). In Nicaragua, prior to 1979, there was no formal provision for deaf children, so they communicated using signs developed within their particular families. After 1979, the government created special schools for deaf children where, spontaneously, the children communicated using their own individual signing systems. This was another example of pidgin, which linguists categorized as Lenguaje de Signos Nicaraguense (LSN). Over time, this pidgin evolved into a Creole, created

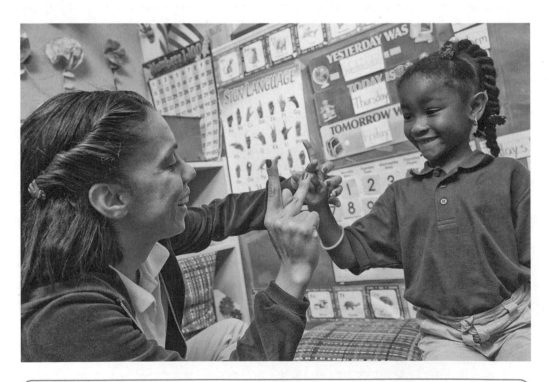

Juan Silva/Getty images

by the younger children who had been exposed to the LSN pidgin of the older children. This evolved into a standardized sign language with grammatical rules, now officially named Idioma de Signos Nicaraguense (ISN). These findings provided further evidence for a universal grammar that underlies all languages.

However, other theorists place much greater emphasis on the interactive social contexts within which children develop pre-linguistic knowledge. Piaget (1936) argued that the child can already communicate with others, long before the first words appear, through gestures, facial expression and actions. Language, according to Piaget, emerges from an existing cognitive system, grounded in sensori-motor experiences. According to Piagetian theory, during the first two years of life, the child's intellectual skills do not rely on symbols, such as words and images, but on sensori-motor experiences, like seeing, hearing and touching. The rules of language, from this perspective, do not come from an LAD but from a much wider cognitive system. Children first form schemas – or systems for explaining the world – to understand events in their lives and afterwards talk about them once they have acquired language. This perspective was very influential but it ignored a crucial aspect of the child's experience – the impact of the social environment on the child's capacity to learn.

Vygotsky (1962) and his followers in social-cultural theory challenged the Piagetian perspective. Vygotsky proposed that it was through the process of reflecting on his/her own thoughts, using language, that the child was enabled to see things in new ways. Vygotsky argued that we can only understand mental functioning by considering it in its social context. He proposed that, at around two years, language begins to overlap with pre-linguistic thought, as represented through gestures, actions and perceptions. From this age, language serves two crucial functions. The first is to monitor internal thoughts; the second is to communicate to others. Children at this age do not distinguish between the two functions and will typically engage in **egocentric speech**, in which the child appears to be thinking aloud. The process of internalizing the thought aspect of language as **inner speech** typically does not come until the child is around 7 years of age when egocentric speech more or less disappears. (In practice, egocentric speech does not entirely disappear since even as adults there are times when we 'think aloud', usually when no one else is there to hear.) Vygotsky's view was that egocentric speech serves the same purpose as inner speech, namely to orient oneself and to come to understand events and interactions in everyday life. Language, from this perspective, mediates between social interaction and cognition throughout development. Children negotiate meanings through discursive interactions, and this process allows for increasing **intersubjectivity**. Thus, social communication is gradually reconstructed as internal speech or 'voices of the mind'. Discourse becomes a social mode of thinking, as indicated later in this chapter in the work of Brown and Renshaw (2000).

Tomasello (2003) complemented the Piagetian and Vygotskian viewpoints by investigating the specific effect of the social environment on the child's capacity to learn language. He proposed that before they begin to talk, children already have a cognitive grasp of the ordering of events in their lives, for example, pushing and pulling, eating, seeing objects move up and down, in and out, things being broken and mended. However, rather than possessing an LAD, he argues, children construct schemas based on their pre-linguistic knowledge in combination with the utterances that they hear in everyday life from adult speakers. On the basis of his observations of children's use of grammatical structures, Tomasello proposed that they move through various stages in their production of language: *holophrases*, *word combinations*, *verb-island combinations* and *adult-like constructions*. For example, 18-month-old children have no difficulty in learning new nouns in combination with words they already know. But they have much more difficulty with verbs. When Tomasello *et al.* (1997) taught 18-month-old children new invented nouns and verbs, such as 'gop' and 'tam', the children were able to use the invented *nouns* flexibly in new contexts (for example, 'two gops!') but were unable to replicate the invented words as *verbs*. For example, despite hearing such sentences as 'It's gopping' from the researchers, hardly any of the children were able to replicate the invented words as verbs, and never used them creatively in tenses that they had not heard ('It gopped!'). On the basis of many experiments testing out children's capacity for making novel word combinations, Tomasello and colleagues concluded that 18–24-month-old children have what they called **pivot grammar**, a form of understanding of the concept of the noun, on which they 'hang' new nouns as they are learned. But at this age, they do not have a similar pivot on which to hang verbs. After 24 months of age, children gradually acquire verb islands, not in the sense of grammatical structures (or an LAD), but rather as schemas that apply to events in their everyday lives. Each verb is developed on a verb-by-verb basis as the child's range of experiences widens and from the child's experience of listening to adult discourse in these situations *before* they are ready to generalize across scenes and events to make grammatical constructions of their own. In other words, from this perspective, the cognitions develop step by step before the child's production of grammar. In order to understand the processes involved, many linguistics experts have turned to the nature of the interactions between adult and child. One fruitful area of enquiry concerns the way in which adults speak to babies, sometimes known as 'motherese' or baby-talk register, but more often now termed infant-directed speech (IDS) and child-directed speech (CDS).

Infant- and child-directed speech

Typically parents/carers speak to their babies in a very special way. This register is currently described as infant-directed speech (IDS) progressing to child-directed speech (CDS). Throughout the history of psycholinguistics, it has been given a range of names, such as baby-talk register and 'motherese' (Saxton, 2010). IDS and CDS are distinct modes of speech. Throughout life, people talk in different registers, depending on the context. For example, the register that a person uses in a formal meeting is different from chat with a close friend in a café. IDS is characterized by exaggerated intonation, rising and falling curves in sound and a higher pitch than usual. IDS is slower, has longer pauses and longer syllables. Babies show preference for this register so it becomes mutually satisfying for both adult and child. Gradually, during the pre-school years, IDS evolves into CDS. Furthermore, as the child's language develops, so CDS adapts in a subtle way throughout childhood and adolescence until it becomes adult-directed speech. Although there are wide differences in the form that it takes, most linguistics experts agree that some form of IDS/CDS is used universally in all cultures, but see the next section for discussion of some disagreement on how to interpret the forms that it takes in different societies. Mithen (2005) notes the highly musical nature of IDS and proposes that infants are very sensitive to the rhythms, tempos and melodies of speech long before they can understand the meaning of the words. As he puts it (ibid.: 72) 'the melody is the message' and he emphasizes the universally musical occurrence of IDS across cultures when adults speak to infants. Furthermore, infants respond with appropriate emotions when listening to speech, whether the language is their own or not, suggesting that they are sensitive to the musical rhythms and tones. In Mithen's (ibid.: 74) words '. . . the mental machinery of IDS belongs originally to a musical ability concerned with regulating social relationships and emotional states'.

Dissanayake (2000) studied the 'microdynamics' of the conversation-like interactions between mothers and their babies. She concluded that each partner in these interactions tracked the emotional expressions displayed in the body, face and voice of the other. In this way, the baby gained a form of emotional regulation that was finely tuned to their immediate level of attention. Dissanayake observed the musical nature of these mutually enjoyable interactions. The musical sounds and rhythms characteristic of IDS appeared to achieve a high level of harmony between the mother and child.

Language and culture

In Western cultures, parents usually nurture the acquisition of words and sentences through myriad rewarding interactions which result in an enormous expansion of language knowledge and use throughout the first five years. From this perspective, the quality of the relationship between caregiver and child is of critical importance, and this has resulted in a great deal of emphasis being placed on the sensitivity of the primary caregiver in facilitating language development. However, as noted in the previous section, it is important to bear in mind that the form of communication styles between parent and child varies widely among cultures. In some cultures there is significantly less emphasis on special 'baby-talk' registers. Schieffelin and Ochs (1998), for example, documented the exchanges between Kaluli (Papua New Guinea) mothers and their infants and found that, in comparison with mothers in Western societies, the Kaluli adults maintained a very clear difference in status between themselves and their infants. In contrast to Anglo-American mothers who typically spend a great deal of time gazing at their babies in face-to-face communication, the Kaluli were more likely to face their babies outward, away from them, so that the babies could see, and be seen by, the social group. When another person spoke to the baby, the mother would often reply for the child in a special high-pitched voice using fully formed adult language. This kind of interaction would not take place until the infant was aged around 4–6 months. Schieffelin and Ochs (ibid.) conclude that, in this Papua New Guinea culture, the process of learning to be social takes place largely through multiple social interactions with the community rather than in the intimacy of the mother-child dyadic communication that is typical of middle-class Western culture.

Research studies tend to confirm the impact that parents' quantity and quality of language has on the fluency and vocabulary of their children. CDS facilitates language development since it is so closely attuned to the child's language needs. There is, however, evidence that there are also wide variations within socio-economic status (SES) bands, as Hurtado *et al.* (2008) found in their study of Spanish-speaking families in disadvantaged communities. Similarly, Hyter and Westby (1996) found that school-aged African-American children demonstrated unique strengths, especially in narrative and poetic uses of language.

A great deal of research has been carried out to investigate the relationship between socio-economic status and language competence. As was indicated in the previous section, individual children have a whole range of experiences of CDS both in terms of quantity and quality. Box 5.1 shows findings from a well-known study by Hart and Risley (1995) which examined differences in everyday language use between parents and children from three contrasting socio-economic contexts: professional parents; working-class parents; and parents on welfare.

Box 5.1

Number of words heard per hour according to socio-economic status (SES) (adapted from Hart & Risley, 1995)

SES of parents	Number of words per hour
Professional	2,153
Working class	1,251
On welfare	616

Here the researchers looked in depth at the quality of the language that took place in the home during verbal interactions between parents and their children. The professional parents were more likely to converse with their children for longer periods of time and to use a wider range of words than the parents on welfare. The researchers found that, by the age of 3 years, children of professional parents were hearing on average 2,153 words per hour in comparison with only 616 words per hour being heard by children of parents on welfare benefits. The children of working class-parents heard on average 1,251 words per hour. Although the children in the lowest SES families heard less talk per hour, they heard more prohibitions (on average 11) than did the children of professional parents (on average 5). So the children from welfare families were told off more often and experienced more negative statements from their parents. In general, high SES parents used longer and more complex utterances with their children, so resulting in wider vocabulary and greater complexity in the child's language. Hart and Risley concluded that children from low-income families were disadvantaged with regard to their language development.

Discussion questions

Is this a valid conclusion or are other interpretations of the quality of language in the home possible? Compare these findings in the light of more recent research on mind-mindedness (see Chapter 2) and the evaluation of Sure Start (see below). What are the implications for children's later achievement in reading and writing?

Efforts to compensate for language deprivation in early life have a long history in the USA, most famously through the Project Headstart initiative (Zigler & Styfco, 2004). The longitudinal evaluation by Lazar and Darlington (1982) demonstrated the general effectiveness of intervention during the early years. Similar positive results have been found in such programmes as The Incredible Years (Webster-Stratton *et al.*, 2008) which emphasize the promotion of social competence as well as language skill.

Most recently, in the UK, intervention includes the Sure Start programme, launched in 1998, a major strategic initiative to end child poverty by changing the ways in which services were delivered to pre-school children and their families, including hard-to-reach groups such as homeless families, and by specifically targeting highly deprived geographical areas in the UK. The Sure Start programme aimed to improve the health and social, emotional and economic development of the children, the health and social, emotional and social development of the parents, and the general well-being of the wider community. The children's linguistic competence was one of the outcomes measured.

A major evaluation by Belsky and Melhuish (2008) found that there were both positive and negative outcomes for children. Thirty-six-month-olds showed fewer behaviour problems, demonstrated greater social competence and greater verbal fluency than those in comparison communities. The adverse effects were among the children of teenage mothers (14% of the sample) who scored lower on verbal ability and social competence and higher on behaviour problems. Children from workless households (40% of the sample) and from lone-parent families (33% of the sample) also showed evidence of adverse effects, such as lower scores on verbal ability. In general, then, the children from *relatively less* disadvantaged families (non-teenage mothers) benefited from the Sure Start intervention while those who were *relatively more* deprived (that is, teenage mothers, workless households and lone parents) did not.

Intersubjectivity and mind-mindedness

There are many factors other than simple measures of SES that support and shape the child's language development. These include the richness of the family's culture, their ethnicity, the presence of bi- or multilingualism and the quality of the attachment that the child has experienced (Hoff, 2006). Cross-cultural research has relevance to the ways in which findings can be interpreted. Though styles of interaction vary across social groups, there remain some very important commonalities. Tomasello *et al.* (2005) argue that a uniquely human ability is the capacity to engage in collaborative activity. This comes very early in the child's life. By 10 months of age, infants can interpret the mother's meaning when she points at an object. This is an early form of shared understanding. Similarly, a child at around the same age can point to something out of reach to indicate that they want it. By 18 months of age, most infants can draw the attention of another person to an object of mutual interest, and to provide some form of commentary about what it is and what the child feels about it.

In all cultures, babies develop in the context of a social group and through participating in communicative activities with members of that society; the infants develop skills, knowledge and mental representations which are all essential for their linguistic growth and their understanding of the concepts that are meaningful in their particular social group. In all societies children enter into what Tomasello (2003) calls an *intersubjective world* when they communicate, whether with their primary caregivers or with members of the wider community. Through this intersubjective process, both adults and children regulate and maintain their interactions with others.

From around 18 months to 36 months of age, the child becomes more 'conversational' and shows awareness that communication need not only be about events in the present but can refer to other shared knowledge. Again, this illustrates the child's growing capacity for developing a theory of mind. Communication is not only tied to immediate events and objects but gradually becomes something of value in its own right. From this point, as Harris (1999:

102) explains, children 'begin to think of people, whether as interlocutors or as agents, as knowers who can take in and retain information that is partial or misleading'. Harris compares these everyday interactions with 'tutorials' in which, over time, the child comes to understand that the people they communicate with have different viewpoints and knowledge. This is at the heart of mind-mindedness and marks the important transition away from egocentric patterns of thought.

Experience of internal-state language continues to be related to children's subsequent understanding of their own and others' internal states (Meins *et al.*, 2006). From around 2 years of age, children themselves start to use words that refer to internal states, whether of perception or emotion. These include such words as 'see', 'want', 'look' and 'taste'. By the age of 3, they can use words like 'think', 'know' and 'remember'. Throughout the pre-school period, language continues to develop rapidly. Frequent communication with peers and adults remains a crucial factor in facilitating the child's capacity to communicate and think (Case Study 5.1). In families where there is a tendency to talk about feelings and what causes them, the children

---

CASE STUDY 5.1

Children demonstrate the capacity to read the minds of others

Jenny tells Izzie that Amy, the cat, has gone up the chimney. Izzie looks worried and stops playing. Jenny laughs and says, 'I was only pretending. You thought Amy went up the chimney. I was just teasing you.'

Jenny shows that she can infer what Izzie is thinking and feeling. She indicates that she understands when another child has a false belief, in this case that Amy has gone up the chimney.

Johnnie, aged 3, says to his friend, Tony, as they are playing with Lego, 'I thought there weren't any yellow bricks left. But then I looked and saw them. They were in your model. I didn't know you had them.'

Johnnie is showing his capacity to distinguish between reality (the yellow bricks are in Tony's model) and belief (he realizes that he was mistaken in thinking that there were no yellow bricks on the table).

Discussion questions

Think of some everyday examples of theory of mind from your own experience of observing children. At what age did these examples occur? Do they confirm theory of mind studies? Think of ways in which you might enhance a child's theory of mind.

are more likely to develop a vocabulary that includes a wide variety of words about their own and others' emotions and perspectives. Parents who more frequently use words that describe emotional states in dialogues with their children demonstrate mind-mindedness which Meins *et al.* (2002) related to enhanced theory of mind skills as well as verbal fluency. This in turn leads the infants to respond more confidently to new experiences, to elicit further affirmative responses from adults around them and so to build on existing linguistic competence. This process is typically done in a playful way and in the context of family events, such as special outings or simply amusing events that occur in the course of everyday life. The child is in this way encouraged to think positively about themselves and their world.

Researchers (e.g., Meins *et al.*, 2006; Ruffman *et al.*, 2002) have devised ingenious experiments to test the links between mothers' use of internal-state language during everyday communication and the child's subsequent understanding of mind. For example, children are asked to describe what they see in a wordless picture book. This tells the story of a pet frog which escapes from his owner, a little boy, and has various adventures. The story contains pictorial information on the characters' emotional reactions to the adventures, including mistaken identity and deception, and provides a range of opportunities for the child to talk about internal feeling states. The child's responses referring to characters' internal states are then categorized. For example: 'she was going to give it to the baby, but the frog got it' was coded as *internal state* because the picture only showed the mother preparing a bottle of milk and the child had to infer that she was intending it for the baby rather than the frog. Again, responses like 'the lady was shocked' indicated that the child was able to infer an emotional state from the pictures. When the child spoke on behalf of one of the story characters in a croaky, frog-like voice ('Mmm, that looks tasty'), this response also indicated awareness of internal states (Meins *et al.*, 2006: 186).

Researchers report a relationship between 3–4-year-olds' use of mental-state language during play with parents/carers and their concurrent theory of mind performance (Nielsen & Dissanayake, 2000). This also extends to conversations that pre-schoolers have with their peers. For example, Brown *et al.* (1996) investigated the frequency of conversational turns that included a mental state reference in interactions between children and their mothers, their siblings and their peers. They found that average mental-state interactions per hour ranged from 2.8 for mother-child conversations, through to 5.1 for child-sibling conversations, through to 13.4 for conversations between a child and a friend. This study indicates how important it is to take account of all the significant people, including other children, with whom the child communicates in everyday life.

A study by Hoff (2010) clearly demonstrates the impact of different types of conversational partner that influence the speech produced by young children (Box 5.2). Hoff recorded the speech of 16 children (8 boys and 8 girls) aged from 21 to 36 months as they played with a sibling aged between 4 and 5 years, a sibling aged between 7 and 8 years and their mother. Hoff measured vocabulary use and grammatical complexity, as well as responses to questions posed by the other speaker. There were significant differences in the language that these young children used depending on the conversation partner. They used a richer vocabulary and answered more questions when they spoke with their mothers than they did with their older siblings, regardless of age. But the grammatical complexity and the number of utterances that they produced were less consistently affected. They were more likely to respond to questions when in conversation with 7–8-year-old siblings than when talking with 4–5-year-old siblings.

Box 5.2

Comparisons of children's speech in 20 minutes of conversation with older siblings and mothers (adapted from Hoff, 2010)

	4–5-year-old sibling	7–8-year-old sibling	Mother
Number of utterances	155.50	175.13	242.05
Number of word types	53.55	50.19	84.50
Mean length of utterance (words)	1.83	1.75	1.72
Responses to questions from conversation partner	5.10	11.81	31.50

This study shows the importance of context and level of support provided by a conversation partner. For example, in asking questions, the mothers probably gave more opportunities for the children to reply than did the older siblings and they appeared to be more attuned to the toddlers' level of competence. Children's speech appears to vary depending on what they are doing and with whom they are interacting.

Discussion question

There are differences in the findings from the studies by Hoff (2010) and from Brown *et al.* (1996) in terms of the relative influence on language production of mothers, siblings and peers. Can you explain why the findings differ?

By the end of the pre-school period, the child should have had a wide range of experiences that prepare for the transition to literacy. For example, they should usually have had experience of singing nursery rhymes and songs, and of listening to an adult read to them and encourage them to comment on the theme of the story. They should have the ability to remember stories that they heard before and have some idea about how to turn the pages of a book to follow the sequences of a narrative. Children at this age also should have some interest in making scribbles to represent letters. It is important for adults to develop storytelling routines with their children from a very early age for a number of reasons (Robbins & Ehri, 1994; Senechal, 1997). The narrative form helps the child: 1) to organize their experiences; and 2) to manage their emotions if they are given plenty of opportunities to do this in the playful context of story. In addition, researchers report that children whose parents regularly tell and retell stories display fewer behavioural and emotional difficulties by the time they get to school age (see Chapters 2 and 3). Children learn to use particular forms of language to signal that they are enacting or telling a story, such as 'Once upon a time' or 'Let's pretend.' By the time that they are around 3 or 4 years of age, children know well how to navigate between the worlds of reality and fantasy by using particular forms of gaze, gesture, tone of voice and posture. At the same time, they are learning about the appropriate language for expressing the hypothetical, for example, by using words like 'if', 'would' and 'might'.

CASE STUDY 5.2

Mark: the language development of a child with Down Syndrome (DS)

Down Syndrome occurs in approximately 1 in 800 live births and is due to a chromosomal abnormality, usually originating in damage to the ovum prior to conception. A woman's ova are present from birth so they are increasingly vulnerable to damage over time, hence, older mothers are more likely than younger mothers to have a baby with DS. Mark's mother, Val, was 42 years old when he was born so she was at higher risk than a younger woman of having a baby with DS. Mark has the specific physical characteristics typical of children with DS, including slanting eyes and an upper eyelid fold. Like most children with DS, Mark is reaching developmental milestones at a later age than is usual. Many children with DS have poor memory for heard speech, delayed speech comprehension and difficulties in pronunciation of words. At the age of 3 years, Mark is still unable to speak.

As indicated in earlier sections of this chapter, research evidence suggests that for most children language and gesture develop alongside one another during the early years. As language evolves, children rely less on gesture to communicate. By contrast, children with DS continue to rely more on gesture than language to communicate than typically-developing children of a similar age. Difficulties in the verbal short-term memory system seem to be a major reason for the speech and language delays in children with DS (Burgoyne, 2009). However, there are a number of interventions that adults can implement to improve short-term memory, for example, through number games that help the child to practice digit span (Conners *et al.*, 2008) and through music training. Ho *et al.* (2003) found that children with DS who had participated in music training between the ages of 1 and 5 years had a better capacity for recalling words than a control group who had not experienced this training. One explanation for this finding is that speech and language development is localized in the left hemisphere of the brain while musical stimuli are processed generally in the right hemisphere. As the child's experience increases, music processing shifts from the right to the left hemisphere. Whatever the reason, the method seems to be successful and it is, at the same time, highly enjoyable for the child.

Val is trying out different games and musical activities to help Mark in this way and he is responding very well. Val is also teaching him **Makaton**, a sign language for children with learning disabilities, and he is responding with great enthusiasm by communicating his needs and wishes to the family in this way.

Mark is very sociable and is keen to relate to other children. He also loves to play with family pets. This interest in peer relationships is likely to continue throughout childhood and adolescence, as indicated by a study of 8–16-year-olds with DS by Begley (1999). He is also attending a playgroup where there are specialist programmes designed to develop play and communication at an early age. Mark has some difficulties with other children at the playgroup but, for the most part, he enjoys the same sorts of activities as other children.

Discussion question

Discuss how best to help Mark to realize his potential through language games and play.

During the pre-school years, children gradually move away from narrating stories through actions so that, by the time they enter first school at the age of around 5 years, their stories are more likely to be expressed in linguistic ways, using dialogue and communication that takes account of the needs of the audience. It is also important to read regularly to children from birth onwards. As the child gets older, they can be encouraged to hold books the right way up, turn the pages as the adult reads and engage with the pictures and text. These are important skills that the child can build on during the school years as they learn to master the principle that letters and sounds go together in a systematic way, become aware of phonetics (the system that governs particular sounds in order to convey meaning), and be able to segment words into their component parts (sounds and syllables). Ways to develop these foundations include:

- Using words to talk about everyday pictures and objects;
- Exploring the shapes, sounds and names of letters and words;
- Using songs to explore rhymes ('the cat sat on the mat', 'Doctor Foster went to Gloucester');
- Playing with alliteration ('each peach pear plum', 'Peter Piper picked a peck of pickled pepper').

As indicated earlier in the chapter, the quality and quantity of the CDS that pre-schoolers have experienced greatly influences the process of making the transition to literacy. From 5 to 8 years of age, children spend a great deal of their time at school learning to read and write. Some of these skills are perceptual. The child needs to take account of visual information as well as the sound and sense of words. Children can be trained to develop these skills through practice in doing jigsaws, matching pictures and shapes, observing similarities and differences, such as 'up', 'down', 'forwards' and 'backwards'. Knowledge of rhyming and alliteration is also essential and this too can be learned in a playful way through nursery rhymes and songs. By learning to play with rhyming sounds they are learning to be aware of speech sounds which lie at the heart of learning to read and spell (Bryant *et al.*, 1990). For example, if the child can read 'beak' this gives him or her a strategy for learning to read a new word 'peak'.

But there are wide variations in the readiness of children for literacy, as discussed in the next section. Helping children to learn to read and write is a very challenging task, particularly if they have not been prepared during the pre-school years.

Making the transition from oracy to literacy

In Western societies, literacy underpins access to education and employment and extends the individual's world from the face-to-face context of verbal communication to a far wider range of experience and knowledge. At the point of beginning formal schooling at around 5 years of age, children are required to make the transition from oracy to literacy. But to do this effectively, they need to have mastered critical pre-reading and pre-writing skills. As Snow (2009: 112) points out, babies are predisposed to speak and to listen. By contrast, reading and writing are social constructs that, first, require specific instruction and, second, build on previous linguistic competence. In order to make a smooth transition to literacy, it is essential that children enter school with a reasonable mastery of pre-reading and pre-writing skills.

There exist different methods for teaching reading and the debate as to which one is most effective continues. Some (e.g., Adams, 1990) place emphasis on the teaching of *phonics* in the context of a meaningful use of text. This approach stresses a logical progression from recognizing individual letters and letter sounds, to sounding out consonant-vowel-consonant words (like 'p-i-g'), to recognizing blends of letters to make new sounds (like 'ch-ip', 'sh-ip' and 'c-ar-t'), to recognizing more complex sounds (like 'igh', 'ou') and split diagraphs (like 'kite' and 'cape'), to alternative sounds (like 'show' and 'frown'), to phonically regular words (like 'cat', 'mat', 'sat') before combining these words into simple sentences (like 'The cat sat on the mat') and into longer texts (like 'Once there was a cat who sat on a mat outside his house'). Bryant and Bradley (1986) and Goswami (1995) argue that phonological awareness underpins success in learning to read. Other reading theorists (e.g., Snowling, 2002) place much more emphasis on reading as a search for meaning. From this perspective, the individual letter sounds and words are best learned in the context of reading longer texts that are interesting and meaningful to the child, in other words, that emphasize the value of semantic skills.

The type of support that is offered to children who are experiencing difficulty in learning to read varies, depending on the underlying theory being adopted at the time (Ireson, 2000; Joliffe, 2004). Some remedial programmes offer highly structured phonics while others focus more on meaningful text reading. There are a number of very effective reading schemes. One that is widely used in the UK is the New Zealand Reading Recovery programme (Clay, 1985) which integrates knowledge of phonics with meaningful use of content. In this programme, children are given many opportunities for speaking and listening as an integral part of learning to read and write. This can be facilitated by encouraging social discourse in the classroom and collaborative learning in which all members of learning groups play an active part. Another successful approach is the Literacy Programme (Hornsby & Shear, 1993) which emphasizes the teaching of phonics in a structured sequence starting with letter sounds before moving on to blending, word reading and spelling, then sentences and finally sentences in texts. Some schools use a mix of methods and combine features of different programmes. However, as Ireson (2000) points out, the type of provision that is available to a child experiencing difficulties in learning to read may depend more on what programme has been adopted in that particular school or local authority rather than on an assessment of that child's particular needs. While

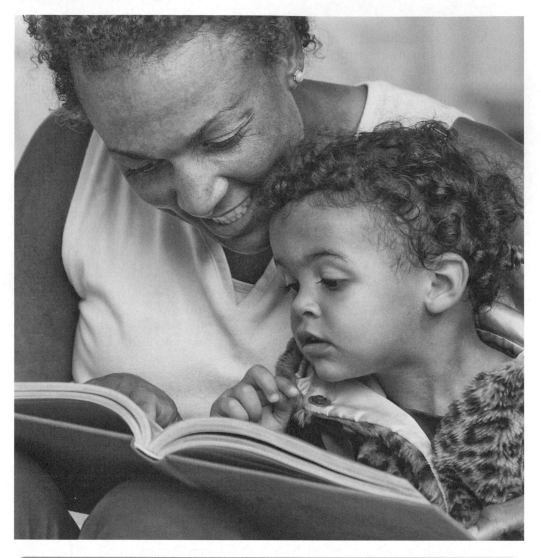

Blend images/Hill Street Studios/Getty images

experienced teachers can adjust their methods to meet the child's needs, novice teachers may find this more challenging

If children have arrived at school with an existing repertoire of pre-reading and pre-writing skills, then most will make a reasonable transition to literacy, though at varying rates of competence. However, those who come to school without full mastery of *oral* skills will lack the psycholinguistic 'tool kit' that facilitates this transition. This will make their life at school increasingly difficult as peers who have mastered reading and writing progress to project work and creative writing. This is a very critical time in the child's school life. Experiencing problems at this stage can underpin later learning, emotional and behavioural difficulties. Expert teaching and support is essential at this stage to give the child the opportunity to catch up (see Case Study 5.3).

Faisal acquires basic pre-reading skills

Faisal was born prematurely and is the youngest of six children, born into a close-knit family where Urdu is the first language. Faisal came from the Reception class to Year 1 with very minimal literacy skills; his Reception class teacher reported that he scarcely spoke to her and had few friends.

On entry to Year 1, his new teacher, Miss Robinson, also noticed that he had poor communication skills, had difficulty in enunciating words and was exceptionally shy, finding if difficult to make eye contact with both adults and other children. He was unable to read at all. With the help of an interpreter, Miss Robinson suggested to his parents that they could help him with reading at home and they agreed that this was a good idea. A selection of sounds on word cards was sent home to facilitate his use of phonics and Miss Robinson also provided some attractive picture books. However, this strategy was not successful. Life at home was hectic, with little time or motivation to act on the suggestion; there appeared not to be any books in the house.

The school had adopted the Reading Recovery method. While the whole class did daily phonics and blends, Faisal was part of a small booster group of six children where the emphasis was on initial sound and letter recognition. He remained in the booster group throughout Year 1. In addition, Faisal was in a daily focus group for literacy run by the classroom assistant as part of the English and Literacy Support scheme. During whole-class lessons, Faisal was also given individual support, either by Miss Robinson or by the classroom assistant.

The issue of literacy support at home was raised again at the next parents' evening, but, although the parents agreed to read to Faisal, in practice they were unable to implement this. Miss Robinson elicited the fact that neither of the parents could read English so she encouraged them to talk about the pictures in the range of easy books which Faisal was taking home each day. The parents appeared to be receptive to this idea and said how much they appreciated the school's efforts, but again very little was done because of family pressures.

The Reading Recovery schemes are graded to allow the child to make progress in simple, small steps. The books are well illustrated. Faisal enjoyed his reading sessions and so his confidence grew. At the same time, his skills in Maths were improving so his self-esteem increased further.

By the end of the year, Faisal was able to maintain eye contact with adults, he began to put his hand up during 'carpet sessions' when children shared their news in a circle, and even volunteered to answer questions during whole-class lessons. His speech became clearer and louder, and he was reading and spelling 'consonant-vowel-consonant' words ('cat', 'bin', 'mat') and becoming more confident with blends ('sh-ee-p', 'sh-i-p').

In Year 2, a similar level of support would be available. Miss Robinson was hopeful that Faisal's progress would continue, provided that daily support was provided.

As was the case in the pre-school years, children continue to respond well to parents'/carers' interest in their daily life at school. This discourse involves more than simply asking what the child did. Rather, it is about genuinely connecting with the child's feelings and experiences, whether of classroom activity or peer relationships. Active listening on the part of adults helps children deal with emotions. Jokes and humour can also help defuse common fears and anxieties. Activities that encourage children's developing literacy from 5 to 8 years of age include: playing word games; asking the child to think of rhymes; asking the child to practice making words out of sounds, for example, 'What words begin with *ba-*?'; asking the child to retell what he/she has just been watching on TV; talking about exciting or funny events from the past; asking the child to think ahead to future events, for example, the party he/she is going to next weekend; encouraging the child to make their own book with their own pictures; looking around in the environment and encouraging the child to read street signs, advertisements, destinations on buses; encouraging the child to write shopping lists.

More advanced activities that support and enhance literacy are an important part of the child's transition from learning to read into reading and writing in order to learn (Snow, 2009). Such activities include:

- *Understanding home and school values* – what is considered to be right and wrong in the family and at school, and why;
- *Understanding societal values* – what are some of the broader issues in society; why some groups are in conflict with others;
- *Developing empathy* – looking at things from different points of view; talking about people's emotions; role-play can be a powerful medium for perspective-taking;
- *Learning to doubt and question* – taking a critical look at what the child hears and reads; having the opportunity to explore controversial issues.

Children at the late primary school stage are also developing a sense of audience. They are learning to adapt their communication style to the type of person that is to hear what they say or read what they write. There are huge opportunities at this stage for the development of citizenship skills and knowledge both through communication in the child's native language and in the process of learning new languages (Starkey, 2005). In discussion work, for example, pupils can learn to listen to one another respectfully, ensure that everyone has a chance to speak, be helpful and constructive when challenging another person's point of view, and positively affirm other pupils when they are helpful and supportive. This in turn has the potential to promote democratic citizenship, as is indicated by one study in Australia using collective argumentation.

An example of the constructive use of language to facilitate thinking and critical skills can be found in the teaching method of *collective argumentation* (Brown & Renshaw, 2000; Schwarz & Linchevski, 2007). Collective argumentation is a form of social exchange that leads to an advance in the participants' knowledge. In this method, children are encouraged to interact with adults and peers through a collective process of discussion, sharing perspectives, presentations of group findings, testing out ideas with other groups in the classroom. The teacher observes, challenges and listens critically to the quality of argumentation at each stage of the process. Brown and Renshaw (2000) found that Australian 10–11-year-olds in classes that practised collective argumentation produced significantly higher levels of verbal interaction than students in control classes that engaged in unstructured open discussion of the same topics. The children made more requests for clarification, justification and elaboration of ideas than in control classes. The larger number of restatements, rephrasings, evaluations and explanations by students indicated that they were working more with one another's ideas rather than with those of the teacher only. In one class, the children developed their own charter of values that incorporated such qualities as: sharing; persistence; patience in waiting turns; respect for others; peer support; honesty; humility. Brown and Renshaw (ibid.) indicate the great value in learning of facilitating the children's capacity for expressing a *voice* and then having that opinion *re-voiced* as an integral part of the collaborative processes at work. By re-voicing what a child says, the teacher assigns authority to that child's viewpoint in a way which can encourage the co-construction of ideas within the learning group. Such exploratory classroom discourse can be developed in any classroom on any topic.

Chapter summary

In this chapter we looked at the main theories of language development. In particular, we considered the crucial role that parents and carers play in their daily communication with children. We examined the concept of mind-mindedness and the adult's concern to treat young children as beings with minds and internal states. Building on this concept, we explored the development of children's pre-reading and pre-writing skills and the importance of reading and telling stories to young children. We also looked at the impact of disadvantaged backgrounds on the development of children's language and communication skills. We looked at the transition from oracy to literacy during the school years, as well as the effectiveness of literacy programmes, and other programmes that enhance critical thinking skills.

Discussion points

- What is the evidence for a universal grammar?
- Why is infant-directed speech so important?
- Can schooling compensate for earlier deprivation in language development?

Further reading

For a very detailed and readable account of child language acquisition, including balanced discussion of the nature-nurture debate, see: Saxton, M. (2010) *Child Language: Acquisition and Development*, London: Sage. For links between language development and music see the highly original book: Mithen, S. (2005) *The Singing Neanderthals*, London: Phoenix. The account of one child's development in the early years also gives fascinating insights into language development in a meaningful context: Fernyhough, C. (2008) *Baby in the Mirror*, London: Granta Books.

Moving forward to the factors that underlie reading difficulties, see: Bryant, P. & Bradley, L. (1986) *Children's Reading Problems*, Oxford: Basil Blackwell, as well as Snowling, M. J. (2002) 'Reading and other learning difficulties', in Rutter, M. & Taylor, E. (eds) *Child and Adolescent Psychiatry*, 4th edition, Oxford: Blackwell Scientific: 682–696.

The resource written by Healthy Schools Derbyshire (2009) *Opening Hearts: Challenging Homophobia and Homophobic Bullying in the Primary School*, Chesterfield, emerging from the Opening Hearts Project, gives invaluable information on the use of teaching literacy in primary schools as a means of challenging homophobic bullying. There is an accompanying CD-ROM and a wealth of materials including poems, narratives, storytelling and theatre scripts.

Websites and resources

Interesting video footage of adult-child interaction from 2 months to 6 years of age in a range of settings:
   www.msu.edu/-casby/langdevidcomp/

The website of the Reading Recovery Council of North America gives useful information on the Reading Recovery programme:
   http://www.readingrecovery.org/reading_recovery/facts/index.asp

See also the University of York website:
   http://www.bestevidence.org.uk/programmes/reading_recovery.html

Similarly, the National Literacy Trust is a useful source:
   http://www.literacytrust.org.uk/

Chapter 6

The impact of traditional and new media

Map of the chapter

Virtually all children and adolescents now watch television and listen to radio; the majority of young people have access to online, mobile and networked media. As children become adolescents, they interact less with parents and more with their peers; the increase in their use of the internet exposes young people to many new contacts well beyond the control of parents. This chapter examines the impact of traditional and new media, including television, video games, advertising and the internet. It explores the benefits, such as information gathering, social networking and leisure pursuits, as well as the risks, such as cyberbullying, exposure to offensive material and manipulation by commercial interests. It ends by outlining current knowledge to enhance safer use of the internet and new online technologies.

The influence of the media

The media and the new technologies have become an everyday part of the lives of young people today. Soon, it is likely that all children and young people will have instant and continuous access to all media, through television, computer games and the internet. While there are huge benefits, there are also risks. So there are important issues to consider with regard to children's emotional, social and cognitive development.

Children and television

From babyhood through to adolescence, television now provides opportunities for children and young people to learn and to expand their horizons. Television offers a diversity of programmes for all ages, featuring news, documentaries, sports and arts performances, nature programmes and child-friendly games and activities. Through this medium, children learn about the logic of narratives, the personal qualities of presenters, cartoon characters and puppets, the conventions of scene-changing, switches in time and location that are typical of television dramas and narratives. They also learn, over time, the difference between fact and fantasy. However, since many programmes are not specifically tailored to meet children's developmental needs, the experience of unsupervised viewing for long periods of time carries risks.

As a result, healthcare professionals and educators have expressed concern about the amount and quality of the television that is offered to children and young people. For example, the American Academy of Pediatrics Committee on Public Education (2001) warned about the dangers of allowing children to have a television set in their bedroom, recommended that pre-schoolers' time watching television should be limited to no more than two hours per day and proposed that children under 2 years should not watch it at all. Instead, parents should encourage interactive activities like talking, playing, singing and reading together that would promote social and cognitive development. Their concern was that children who watched too much television would suffer later in terms of educational achievement (see also Byron, 2008; Evans Schmidt *et al.*, 2008). Furthermore, if adults were not selective about guiding viewing choice, the child might be exposed to material that was upsetting or even damaging.

At the same time, the media were producing educational programmes, such as *Sesame Street,* which currently broadcasts to over 100 million children in 150 countries, with the aim of engaging pre-schoolers in activities such as: learning new words, understanding basic mathematics, recognizing colours and shapes, dealing with social and emotional issues, solving conflicts. There is continuing debate about the educational value of television for children. In the UK, for example, such programmes as *In the Night Garden* and *Teletubbies* appeal directly to toddlers through the use of the simplified sentence structure and the repetition of one- and two-word phrases that are typical of this age group. Viewers watch a series of familiar routines portrayed by the characters, for example, television screens portrayed on the *Teletubbies'* stomachs repeating short documentaries on topics of interest to the very young. Some critics have criticized such programmes on the grounds that regular viewing of *Teletubbies* can actually delay children's language development. Box 6.1 reports on research that defuses some of the controversy about the educational value of television.

Box 6.1

Learning from *Teletubbies* (adapted from Marsh, 2003)

Marsh (2003) investigated the responses of young children to *Teletubbies* in three primary schools and two nurseries in inner-city areas, using field notes, photographs, children's work and interviews with staff. She reported on the children's responses to enlarged Teletubby comics during literacy lessons:

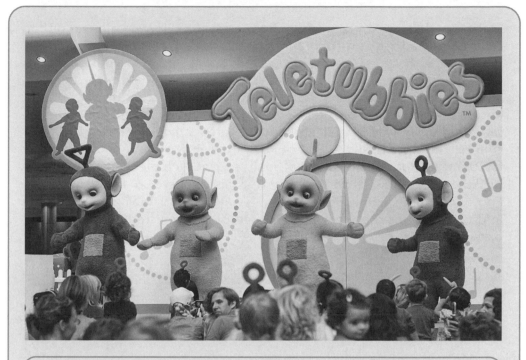

Ian Gavan/Stringer/Getty images

As soon as Jane placed the comic on the big-book stand, there was a wave of excitement from the class and whispers of 'Teletubbies comic!' Jane discussed the layout of the front of the comic with the children and the interchange demonstrated that they were very confident with the genre. The shared reading of the story contained within the comic was obviously enjoyed by all and children maintained interest throughout, demonstrating familiarity with the characters and ability to predict key sequences. This was especially noticeable with children who were in the early stages of acquiring English, children who were not usually able to sustain concentration throughout a shared reading session.

(ibid.: 3)

Some children sustained more interest in the writing activities based on the *Teletubbies* than writing activities based on other topics. For example, Yassar, a 5-year-old child, asked to take part in almost every writing activity based on the *Teletubbies* comics. He was not usually, according to the class teacher, so vociferous in his requests to write . . . It was his love of the *Teletubbies* which was the key to his motivation.

(ibid.: 4)

Marsh concludes that programmes like *Teletubbies* provide motivation for children to read and write (e.g., writing recipes for 'tubby custard'). She also recommends that nurseries and schools should build on the skills that children are acquiring through televisual print encountered on TV screens, computers and video games. She argues that educators need to recognize the positive impact of technology on literacy practices as we move into the 'media-saturated environment' that surrounds children as an integral part of their culture. This research shows that children from all backgrounds benefit from watching *Teletubbies* provided that adults engage with the children and build on what they learn from viewing (see also Roberts & Howard, 2005). Educational programmes designed in this way for pre-schoolers are especially important for the cognitive development of children from disadvantaged backgrounds.

Discussion question

Do you agree that programmes like *In the Night Garden* and *Teletubbies* have educational value?

The impact on children of viewing violence on television

There is also evidence of a link between time spent watching violent programmes on television and later aggression. In an early study, Lefkowitz *et al.* (1977) found the effects were most pronounced for boys. Those who liked to watch violent television programmes at age 9 were significantly more likely to be rated by their peers as aggressive by age 19. This study continued until the participants were 30 years old (Eron, 1987) and the follow-up findings confirmed the trend. Those who liked to watch violent television at 9 years of age were more likely to have criminal convictions as adults. Of course, there are many other factors involved in a child's life besides their choice of television programme so these findings must be taken in context and over time.

Huesmann (2007) has been investigating aggression in television, cinema and video games for over a decade. He distinguishes between short-term and long-term effects of exposure to media violence, as well as *time-displacement effects*, that is, the role of the mass media in displacing other activities in which children might otherwise be engaged, such as reading or taking part in sports. With regard to short-term effects, he identifies the following key processes:

● *Priming* is the process through which activation in the brain's neural network from an external locus (in this case a violent TV programme) excites another brain node representing a cognition, emotion or behaviour. The primed concepts make behaviour linked to them more likely. So the experience of watching characters on TV behaving aggressively stimulates aggressive behaviour in children.

- *Arousal* occurs when a stimulus (such as an exciting media presentation) leads to less inhibition of inappropriate responses and to the display of dominant learned responses, such as direct aggression.
- *Mimicry* takes place when children observe violent behaviour and then enact it in their everyday lives.

With regard to long-term effects, Huesmann identifies three further processes:

- *Observational learning:* Children's beliefs are influenced by their observation of the behaviours of those around them, including those observed in the mass media. Extensive viewing of violence can lead to a distortion in their perceptions of others and result in the attribution of hostility to others' actions, even when none exists. So, repeated observation of characters behaving aggressively on TV changes children so that they behave more aggressively in real life in the long term.
- *Desensitization:* Long-term socialization effects of exposure to violence in the media can lead to a process of *desensitization* whereby the child becomes habituated to scenes of violence. They lack empathy for others' suffering and so can inflict pain on others without feeling any remorse.
- *Acting out what they see:* Children also play an active part in media interactions, for example, when they act out scenes observed in television dramas. So, they may find it enjoyable and rewarding to behave aggressively.

Knowledge of these processes, in Huesmann's view, should guide educators' work in developing interventions to counteract online aggression. Huesmann's research also extends into children's use of video games.

Video games

Many children enjoy playing computer games, such as Xbox. Games give children a sense of control and mastery; there are opportunities to identify with particular characters and the graphics are designed to appeal to children. With developments in virtual reality, narrative approaches in game-playing involve extensive interactivity since the players can actively engage with the characters, the plots and the environment in the game. There is evidence that game-playing enhances children's spatial ability, their attention span and their capacity for logical reasoning (Green & Bavelier, 2006). Some games, such as Wii, require physical activity and can be used in schools to encourage greater involvement in sports and physical education (Physical Education Teachers' Exergaming Resource, 2010).

However, there are risks, as we saw in the section on television viewing. In the USA, 90% of children aged from 8 to 16 years play video games at home, of which most contain violent scenes. The violence includes graphic images of bloodshed and characters that deliberately harm others. As Huesmann (2007) found, playing a violent game causes an immediate rise in aggressive behaviour and aggressive emotions. Similarly, a large meta-analysis of 136 studies from Western and Eastern cultures (Anderson *et al.*, 2010) found that excessive use of violent video games was associated with aggressive behaviour and with a corresponding reduction in empathy for others' feelings and lower expression of prosocial behaviour (Box 6.2).

Box 6.2

Longitudinal effects of violent video games on aggression in Japan and the USA (adapted from Anderson *et al.*, 2008)

In three independent longitudinal studies, the researchers examined children's video game habits and physically aggressive tendencies at two time points, separated by 3 to 6 months. The first sample consisted of 181 Japanese students aged from 12 to 15 years, the second sample of 1,050 Japanese students aged from 13 to 18 years, and the third sample of 364 US students aged from 9 to 12 years. The researchers found that those young people who habitually played violent video games were significantly more likely to be physically aggressive. This study confirmed earlier work and indicated that the longitudinal effect generalized across cultures. It also showed that, relative to those young people who did not play violent video games often, the habitual users had a heightened risk of aggressive behaviour. The effect was more pronounced in the younger children in these samples.

Discussion question

How worried should parents be about allowing their children to play virtual games unsupervised?

An early warning was sounded by Newson (1994) who produced an influential report on the topic of video violence and its impact on young people. She argued that children in Western society were being damaged by the preponderance of violent images and themes in videos. Most recently, the Byron Review (Byron, 2008) examined the potential risk to children of video and internet games. While acknowledging that they offer many opportunities for enjoyment and learning, Byron expressed concern that some of the content is extremely violent. Her proposals include the following recommendations:

- There should be a shared culture of responsibility with regard to internet games;
- Families, industry, government and others in the public domain should collaborate in order to reduce the availability of violent material to children;
- The current classification system should be reformed in order to raise awareness of content in the games and to enable more effective enforcement.

To this end, new games with an educative purpose are evolving that build on children's interest in this medium. They are designed in an emotionally intelligent way so that the games deliberately engage the players in considering the outcomes of certain behaviours and the impact on characters' emotions (Box 6.3).

Educational virtual learning environments (VLEs): the FearNot! programmes (adapted from Aylett *et al.*, 2005; Hall *et al.*, 2006; Watson *et al.*, 2007)

One way forward comes from innovative virtual learning environments (VLEs) that educate children in ways of counteracting bullying with such programmes as FearNot!, an acronym for Fun with Empathic Agents to Reach Novel Outcomes in Teaching. These prosocial programmes have the potential to challenge educators' and parents' understandable concerns about the violence that is often portrayed on commercial DVDs and computer games. The FearNot! method provides 8–11-year-old children with the opportunity to explore a virtual school environment complete with bullies, victims, by-standers, assistants to the bully and defenders of the victim. Participants in the game witness a bullying episode and then 'talk to' the victim characters in order to advise them about what to do next. For example, if a child advises a character to hit the bully back, many different narrative outcomes are possible. Children enjoy the opportunity to try out different methods for dealing with aggressive behaviour in a safe environment. The cartoon meta-phor is one that most children engage with naturally.

Discussion question

How appealing would these games be to children and young people in comparison with Xbox?

Advertising directed at children

Children are a major market for certain products, including clothes, toys, food, drinks and entertainment. They are exposed to thousands of advertisements every year, including advertise-ments directed specifically at them. This has raised concerns that advertising encourages children to be materialistic, an issue which can lead to conflict between parents and children. Another concern relates to the quality of products aimed at children and whether they actually benefit or harm them. Advertisers invest money and effort in their attempts to influence children to buy their goods. But there is growing concern that advertising is unfair if it targets young people in order to promote products that are actually harmful, particularly at an age when children are not aware of the persuasive powers of the advertisers.

At what age do children understand that they are being persuaded to desire certain products? As Ali *et al.* (2009) point out, from about the age of 5–6 years children realize that television advertisements are a source of information, for example, about where to buy certain toys, but they do not appreciate that the information provided in this way has the intention of persuading viewers to buy a product. By the age of 7 or 8 years children are aware of the persuasive nature of television advertisements. The American Psychological Association Task Force on Advertising and Children (2004) argued that media literacy training alone would not be sufficient to protect young children from unscrupulous advertising in the light of their cognitive limitations, although they accepted that older children, from the age of 7 years onwards, could benefit from such efforts.

One example is the large amount of advertising for unhealthy drinks and snacks which may be a strong factor contributing to the rise of **obesity** in children. (For example, in 2008, the UK government banned advertising of food that is high in fat, salt or sugar.) Ali *et al.* (2009) took the issue one step further in their investigation of the age at which children can identify advertisements on a web page, since increasingly manufacturers embed advertisements into web pages designed for children, complete with activities and games. They showed 6–12-year-olds printed versions of invented web pages that included typical internet advertisements and asked them to identify the advertisements. Whereas previous researchers had found that children correctly identify television advertisements from the age of 5 or 6 years, Ali and colleagues found that children were significantly less able to identify advertisements on the internet. As you can see in Box 6.4, 6–8-year-old children were not good at distinguishing advertisements and other content on web pages; 10–12-year-olds were more successful but only identified about three-quarters of the advertisements. This was in contrast to their higher ability to distinguish accurately between TV commercials and programmes.

Box 6.4

Percentage of children who correctly identify advertisements embedded in web pages in the UK and Indonesia (adapted from Ali *et al.*, 2009)

Age	UK (%)	Indonesia (%)
6 years	28	32
8 years	46	54
10 years	73	70
12 years	Data not gathered	78

This research raises worrying issues since it indicates that even at 12 years of age a large proportion of children are not aware of what is factual content and what is a marketing message. Companies can now communicate directly to children through the new media, so resulting in even greater risks to children.

Discussion question

To what extent should the marketing companies be directly challenged on this form of advertising?

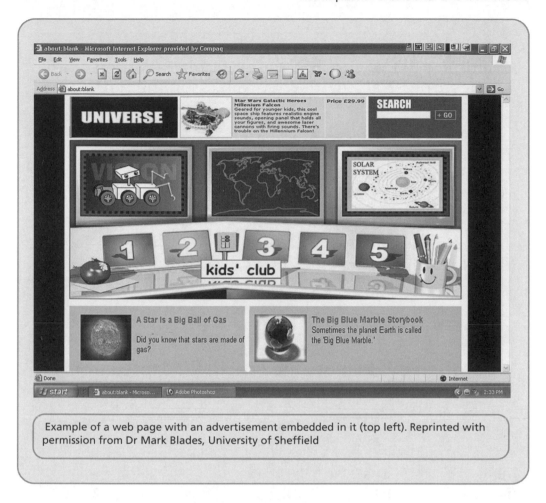

Example of a web page with an advertisement embedded in it (top left). Reprinted with permission from Dr Mark Blades, University of Sheffield

There are examples of possible strategies to overcome this risk. For example, Pempek and Calvert (2009) indicate that it is possible to counteract what they call the obesity crisis among children in the USA, particularly among those from low-income families where the risk is highest. They suggest that the internet could be used proactively to promote healthy eating through the use of **advergames** in order to alter children's eating habits in favour of more nutritious foods. **Advergaming** is the practice of using video games to advertise a product, organization or viewpoint. As we saw, the method is often used by major companies to promote a new product. By focusing on activities that children enjoy, such as playing online advergames, online social marketing approaches could become a cost-effective method to help address the obesity crisis.

Children and the internet

Children are discovering diverse ways of going online, many of which are not supervised by adults. The average age at which children first go online is between 7 and 9 years. In the UK, 49% of children and young people between the ages of 9 and 16 years use the internet in their own bedrooms at home; 47% use it at home but not in their own bedroom (Box 6.5). A breakdown of internet usage by age across Europe is shown in Box 6.6.

Box 6.5

Children's use of the internet at home (adapted from Livingstone *et al.*, 2010, www.eukidsonline.net)

	At home in own bedroom (%)	At home but not in bedroom (%)
Girls	46	38
Boys	50	36
All children	48	37
9–10-year-olds	29	55
11–12-year-olds	43	39
13–14-year-olds	52	32
15–16-year-olds	67	22

Box 6.6

How often children use the internet (adapted from Livingstone *et al.*, 2010, www.eukidsonline.net)

	Every day (%)	Once or twice a week (%)	Once or twice a month (%)	Less often (%)
Girls	55	37	6	3
Boys	60	33	6	2
All children	57	35	6	2
9–10-year-olds	33	52	10	5
11–12-year-olds	51	40	6	3
13–14-year-olds	66	29	6	3
15–16-year-olds	77	20	3	1

Discussion question

Box 6.5 shows that most adolescents access the internet at home and in the privacy of their own bedrooms, rather than in the more public areas of the home. In Box 6.6 you can see how often children and young people of different ages go online. Should parents be concerned about the risk of becoming addicted to the internet?

Social networking is one of the fastest-growing media among young people, involving chat, messaging, making contacts, displaying photo albums and blogging. Sixty-five per cent of children in the UK aged between 11 and 16 years report that they have a profile on a social networking site, and 27% admit to putting an incorrect age on their profile. Most children use the internet safely and with enjoyment, and the vast majority of children report satisfaction with the quality and relevance of the materials that they encounter online (Livingstone *et al.*, 2010).

There are huge benefits to children offered by the internet through shared personal computers, laptops, TV, mobile phones and games consoles. The benefits include:

- New opportunities for learning;
- Games and play;
- Participation in online communities;
- Creativity;
- Widespread communication and access to information.

These diverse communication media offer new approaches to learning. For example, in some classrooms children are given opportunities to create virtual story-worlds that extend literacy by building on children's access to the new media. Box 6.7 shows how some teachers are developing innovative methods for facilitating children's learning to critique materials, look at ideas from different perspectives, develop awareness of their culture and that of others, and to think constructively about contemporary issues.

Box 6.7

Bringing the new media into the classroom (adapted from Waller, 2010)

In this film-making project, primary school children selected a Japanese text, *Kiki's Delivery Service* by Eiko Kadono, which was available as a picture book and anime film by Studio Ghibli. The story is about an apprentice witch, Kiki, who moves to a new town and sets up a delivery service using her broomstick. The children engaged in activities that immersed them in Kiki's world through character profiling, drama activities, illustration and retelling of the story. They then looked at the narrative and how it related to other texts, such as Western fairy tales. The children then discussed how to adapt the Japanese text for a Western audience. This led to a shared narrative where Kiki delivered items to Cinderella, Peter Pan, the Little Mermaid and the Billy Goats Gruff. Then the children created their own virtual world using digital technology by drawing their own backgrounds of the settings then using 'green-screen' techniques to appear in front of them on-screen. The result was an impressive cross-cultural narrative which blended children's knowledge and interpretations of story settings within a virtual space. So the children in this project designed their own virtual world while learning key literacy skills.

Discussion question

To what extent might educational projects like this strengthen the capacity of children and young people to be critical of the media?

Risks from the internet

However, in parallel with adult worries about excessive television viewing, there are current anxieties about the ways in which the internet dominates children's attention. First, there are realistic concerns about the sheer amount of time spent online and the extent to which this crowds out other important activities, such as doing school work, being with family and socializing face-to-face with friends. In many families, the children use the internet more than their parents, a phenomenon which can make it extremely difficult for parents to monitor what their children are doing online or which sites they are visiting. The greatest concerns centre on the management of what is 'private' and what is 'public', and on the potential risks around age verification, cyberbullying, harassment and communication of inappropriate material. Children and young people often seem to be unaware of the permanence of the information that they upload onto the internet and of the difficulties involved in removing compromising or embarrassing photographs, video clips and blogs or abusive materials.

CASE STUDY 6.1

A young person is disturbed by unsolicited sexual images

Letter to a teenage magazine:

Me and my friend were on the computer together when we accidently clicked on this link that was for this inappropriate website. The first thing that came on the screen was these two people having sex. We quickly went off it of course, but I can't get the image out of my head! It is just there, and it has been for about two weeks! I'm scared it might never go away! Please help me. Anon

Discussion question

How would you help this young person?

Common risks include the following:

- Being bullied;
- Encountering pornography;
- Sending or receiving sexual messages ('sexting');
- Meeting offline with people first encountered online.

As Box 6.8 indicates, a proportion of children and young people have seen sexual images online. Of those, nearly half are upset by the experience, with the younger age groups expressing the greatest distress.

Box 6.8

Seeing sexual images online (adapted from Livingstone *et al.*, 2010, www.eukidsonline.net)

	Seen sexual images on the internet (%)	Upset out of those who had seen such images (%)
Girls	12	43
Boys	15	32
9–10-year-olds	6	58
11–12-year-olds	9	47
13–14-year-olds	17	36
15–16-year-olds	24	29

Discussion questions

How can society protect children and young people from unsolicited sexual images? Should the internet providers be doing more to prevent these images from being circulated?

Cyberbullying

Another risk arises from cyberbullying, which refers to a form of covert psychological bullying using electronic devices such as e-mail, mobile phones, text messages, video clips, instant messaging, photos and personal websites in order to engage in repeated hostile behaviour intended to harm another person or persons. It also includes cyberstalking, harassment, denigration and exclusion, teasing or making unpleasant comments online.

Smith *et al.* (2008) surveyed 533 secondary school students and found that the incidence figures for being cyberbullied were as follows:

- 6.6% often (two or three times a month, once a week or several times a week);
- 15.6% only once or twice;
- 77.8% never.

Cyberbullying increased with age and the most reported types of cyberbullying were instant messaging (9.9%), telephone calls (9.5%) and text messages (6.6%). These findings are broadly in line with the results of a large population study of 2,215 Finnish adolescents aged 13–16 years (Sourander *et al.*, 2010) in which the researchers found that 4.8% were cybervictims only, 7.4% were cyberbullies only and 5.4% were cyberbully-victims. These findings indicate that cyberbullying and cybervictimization are less prevalent than traditional bullying or victimization. Traditional victims tended to be cybervictims and traditional bullies tended to be cyberbullies; additionally, traditional bully-victim status was associated with all cyberbully and cybervictim groups. These findings confirm other studies that indicate links between online and offline bullying. Some cybervictims suffer acute emotional distress. Sourander *et al.* (ibid.) found that:

- Nearly 1 in 4 cybervictims reported feeling unsafe;
- These children were more likely to have psychosomatic problems, such as headaches, recurring abdominal pain and sleeplessness;
- They also had peer relationship difficulties.

Cyberbullies also reported emotional difficulties:

- They felt unsafe at school;
- They felt unsupported by their teachers;
- They had a high incidence of headaches;
- They had high levels of conduct disorders and hyperactivity;
- They engaged in frequent smoking and alcohol consumption;
- They had low scores for prosocial behaviour.

The most vulnerable of all were those children who were both cyberbullies and cybervictims. This is in line with studies of traditional bully-victims who tend to be most strongly at risk of a wide range of psychological problems, crime and suicidal thoughts. Research findings on the mental health risks related to cyberbullying indicate the need to create clear guidelines for healthy, prosocial behaviour on the internet. In the next section, we describe action that is currently taking place in this domain.

Young people now have the power to exclude peers from social networks by means of e-mail or text messaging, often in the context of the group or gang (Jones *et al.*, 2011). This phenomenon has a huge impact on our understanding and treatment of communication and relationship difficulties in childhood and adolescence (Snow, 2009). As you can see in Box 6.9, children and young people are capable of sending extremely nasty messages by text with the deliberate intention to hurt and humiliate the recipients. Internet bullying can also involve threats of physical violence or death to a person or their family, or psychological bullying such as posting offensive and embarrassing material about a person on a website, or menacing chain messages.

Box 6.9

Ten categories of offensive text message received by children (adapted from Rivers & Noret, 2010)

- Threat of physical violence: *'I'm going to kick your head in'*;
- Abusive or hate-related: *'I h8u'*; *'You f***ing clown-faced b*****d'*;
- Name-calling (including homophobia): *'Lesbian'*; *'u r gay'*;
- Death threats: *'Trust me you're gonna die bitch'*;
- Ending of platonic relationships: *'You are a slag I'm never gonna speak to you again'*;
- Sexual acts: *'I want to f*** you'*;
- Demands: *'Get me 10 packets of polos, chuddy'*;
- Threats to damage existing relationships: *'I'm going to tell him that you said . . .'*;
- Threats to home/family: *'I will get you and your family too'*;
- Menacing chain messages: *'Send this message to ten of your friends. If you don't you will pay!'*; *'I am going to infect your computer with a virus'*.

Discussion questions

What power does the peer group have to prevent such unpleasant text messages? How can adults intervene to address the issue?

Jones *et al.* (2011) investigated children's reactions to unpleasant text messages and found that group membership increased the intensity of emotions felt in relation to a bullying incident. The extent to which an individual child identified with the group deeply affected their responses to a bullying incident. One striking finding was that if an individual was strongly affiliated with the group, then he or she was more likely to feel pride in the perpetrator's bullying actions. If a group has a reputation for unkind behaviour and acts in accordance with it, then greater pride in the perpetration of bullying was felt by the group's members. In the absence of such norms, individual children tended to feel less pride in actions that are hurtful to another child. In other words, the group has a very powerful influence on the emotions that children experience when they are involved in unkind communications such as offensive text messaging. In turn, the group influences individual children's actions in such situations, for example, whether to condone being a witness of such communication or whether to intervene to prevent them.

Sanctions and the law

The UK government has linked together committees that are knowledgeable about e-safety, child protection online and bullying both offline and online. Extensive governmental action has taken place through the work of the UK Council for Child Internet Strategy (UKCCIS). The government commissioned the Byron Review (Byron, 2008) which recommended that a priority focus of UKCCIS should be the development of a more effective regulation framework to build on best practice, to promote transparency and to provide families with the tools and reassurance they need for their children, as can be seen in Box 6.10.

Box 6.10

Recommendations of the Byron Review (Byron, 2008)

The Byron Review recommended that:

- There should be an independently monitored voluntary code of practice on the moderation of user-generated content;
- Providers should be committed to removing offensive material;
- There should be moves to clarify the law on certain types of offensive online material;
- The internet industry should actively promote responsible advertising to children online;
- Search providers should give users the option to lock in safe search settings;
- There should be clear links to child safety information from search pages;
- There should be a review of good practice on age verification;
- There should be awareness of changing risks to children from mobile internet access.

Discussion question

How far have these recommendations been adopted in the years since the review was published?

As a result, UKCCIS has devised a range of interventions and policies to improve the e-safety knowledge and skills of children, young people and parents. It also promotes a National Acceptable Use Policy toolkit for all schools, referencing responsible use of school IT networks and equipment, VLEs and mobile phones. The Media Literacy Task Force (2009) proposed that the most effective way of ensuring e-safety was to ensure that adults and children are media literate.

The Education and Inspections Act (2006) includes legal powers relating to cyberbullying and the powers that head teachers have to regulate the conduct of pupils when they are off-site, including the issue of confiscating mobile phones and other items. Cyberbullying is not a specific criminal offence, but there are criminal laws that can apply in terms of harassment, and threatening and menacing communications. The message that inappropriate behaviour online can potentially be a criminal act is one that urgently needs to be communicated to the public at large.

As indicated by UK Internet Security Report (2009) one of the most difficult challenges is convincing people that internet crime is a reality. The same report notes that the very language of cybercrime – terms such as 'phishing' or 'hacking' – gives the impression that online crime is unrelated to real life. It is essential to convince people that behaviour online can have the same impact on others as that same behaviour would have in real life. As the authors of the report point out, '. . . personal attacks, including bullying or using social networking for criminal purposes, can destroy lives whether online or offline'. They conclude that, by working with international law enforcement partners, it is possible to share intelligence, knowledge, tools and techniques in order to catch and, if possible, prosecute perpetrators. The advice offered by the Get Safe Online initiative is that we must all take responsibility for protecting ourselves and those close to us. In the specific context of cyberbullying among children and young people, this adds weight to the view that schools have a critical role to play in educating students to behave responsibly online.

Conclusion

The information and communications technologies (ICTs) have become a major part of children's lives for the purposes of entertainment, seeking information and interacting with peers. For adolescents, ownership of a mobile phone is almost universal. They also use personal computers, games consoles and MP3 players. However, access to ICT is affected by level of family income, with those young people from disadvantaged homes being less likely to have home ownership of a personal computer and broadband. The vast majority of children and young people use the internet in positive ways. But, as there is also the potential for psychological and social damage, adults need to remain vigilant. Children need to be with other people in order to develop their language and communication skills. Furthermore, they need to take regular part in creative play and problem-solving, as well as physical activity that provides opportunities for fresh air and exercise. (As indicated in Chapter 7, children who spend too much sedentary time at a screen run the risk of childhood obesity.)

When the child is engaged with ICT, it is important for the adults to be involved in the computer activities and games that interest their child. For example, the adult can play games with the child and encourage the child to talk about what is on the screen, rather than passively accept it. Adults can also encourage children to be critical and questioning about the material they encounter in the media and online, particularly with regard to information.

Chapter summary

Watching television: Television can play an important part in the child's development and has widespread educational influence. However, adults need to engage with children's viewing and play an active part in using the medium of television to extend children's horizons, develop their vocabulary, enhance speaking and writing skills and understand conventions of narrative. Adults also need to protect children from unhelpful influences, such as the manipulation of children's tastes for commercial advantage.

Computer games: Most children enjoy playing computer games and often engage with games socially with members of their peer group. Games can also be used for educational and physical exercise purposes. However, there are some risks, especially where the content is excessively violent. As with television, adults need to monitor and supervise if possible the extent to which their children use these games and the impact that violent content potentially has on them.

Access to the internet: Younger children from the age of around 7 years generally access the internet in public areas of the home, but as they get older they tend to use the internet in the privacy of their bedrooms. This means that adults need to be proactive if they are to supervise and monitor effectively their children's activity online. It is advisable to start while the child is young by engaging in regular conversations about online activity and ensuring that children are aware of e-safety practices. Adolescents are more likely than younger children to encounter risks, such as cyberbullying or viewing pornographic material, but they are more equipped to deal with the risks, for example, by deleting or blocking sites or by confiding in a peer. The younger children who do encounter adverse material online, however, are more likely to be distressed by it, so adults need to be alert to this danger.

Restrictions: Government can legislate to restrict children's television viewing and providers can block inappropriate material, including advertisements that encourage unhealthy eating. But this also depends on the active involvement of parents to monitor their children.

Co-viewing: Parents are advised to show an interest in their children's use of the new media and to facilitate discussions about what is being viewed and downloaded. As with television viewing, they are advised to engage with their children's activity online and use it as a basis for discussion about critical issues and sharing of experiences.

Media literacy: Many children and young people are going online without the necessary knowledge of e-safety. Adults involved with children are advised to teach e-safety skills and knowledge.

Discussion points

- Why do some health and education experts recommend that parents/carers should limit children's television viewing time? What are the potential dangers? Are there any benefits?
- Do violent video games cause children to become more aggressive? What is the evidence to back up your point of view?
- How can adults protect children and young people from being cyber-bullied?

Further reading

For a useful overview of research into media violence, see: Kirsch, S. (2006) *Children, Adolescents and Media Violence*, Thousand Oaks, CA: Sage. See also: Livingstone, S., Haddon, L., Gorzig, A. & Olafsson, K. (2010) *Risks and Safety on the Internet*, London: London School of Economics. Download from: www.eukidsonline.net

For an up-to-date review of the literature on young people's online communication and the use of the internet for forming and maintaining relationships, see: Mesch, G. & Talmud, I. (2010) *Wired Youth: The Social World of Adolescence in the Information Age*, London: Routledge.

Websites and resources

To see children working creatively with the new media, view YouTube film, *Engage Me*, made by the pupils of Robin Hood Primary in Birmingham:
 http://www.youtube.com/watch?v=s1YoCx384GQ

The ESRC Seminar series, *Children's and Young People's Digital Literacies in Virtual Online Space*, Seminar 5 – *Virtual Literacies in Schools*, can be downloaded from:
 www.changinghorizons.net

The Byron Review provides a comprehensive overview of the online risks that young people face today:
 http://www.dcsf.gov.uk/byronreview/

Similarly, Linda Papadopoulos reviews the sexualization of young people:
 www.homeoffice.gov.uk/documents/Sexualisation-young-people.pdf

The Anti-bullying Alliance (ABA) website provides up-to-date information on cyberbullying:
 http://www.anti-bullyingalliance.org.uk/

For a website designed by WiredKids to provide information for parents and young people about cyberbullying and how to prevent it see:
 http://www.stopcyberbullying.org

CyberTraining is a European project with training materials for parents/carers, teachers, healthcare professionals and young people to use to counteract cyberbullying:
 http://cybertraining-project.org/

Chapter 7

Addictions, obesity and eating disorders

Map of the chapter

This chapter begins by examining the health risks that arise from excessive consumption of alcohol, drugs and other substances. It goes on to examine challenges that arise from the rising incidence of overweight and obesity in childhood and adolescence, health risks from excessive dieting, and major eating disorders, including anorexia nervosa and bulimia nervosa.

Alcohol and the use of drugs

Alcohol is an important part of UK youth culture, as it is in the adult population where alcohol consumption is widespread. Young people drink for a variety of reasons: perhaps to reduce anxiety in social situations or simply to be part of the peer group; to change mood; to deal with stress; to feel happy and sociable with friends; to explore sexual relationships; to provide an excuse or outlet for antisocial behaviour. Young people initially drink at home or in friends' houses and, as they get older, the venue shifts to public spaces, parties and clubs, and finally to pubs.

Of concern is hazardous drinking – that is, drinking associated with the risk of physical or psychological harm. In the last 20 years, hazardous drinking (for example, excessive binge drinking in order to get drunk) among UK youth has become the worst in Europe, resulting in increased risk of accidents, injuries and related illnesses (Gunning & Nicholson, 2010). In England in 2008/2009, 7,537 young people under the age of 16 accessed treatment for alcohol use (National Treatment Agency for Substance Misuse, 2010). Substantial numbers of children and young people drink weekly at risky levels, with an estimated 630,000 11–17-year-olds drinking twice or more each week (Donaldson, 2009).

Currie *et al.* (2008) found two disturbing trends in the drinking patterns of young people:

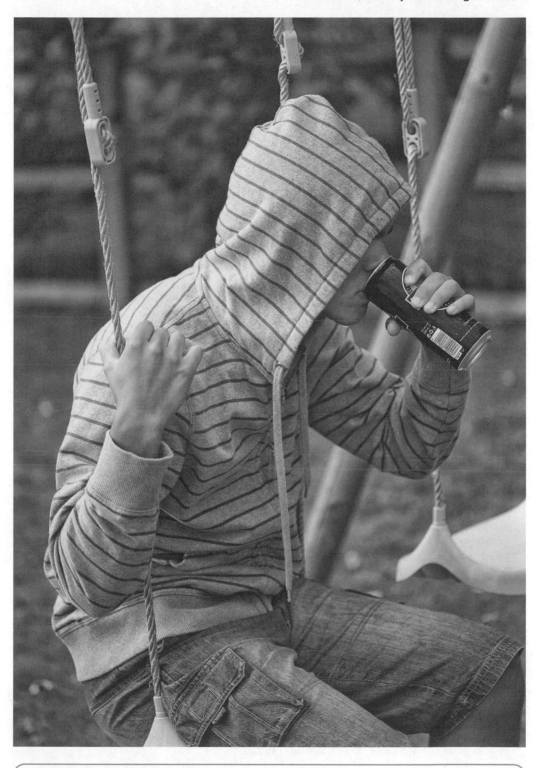

GSO Images/Getty images

- The increase in drinking levels among younger teenagers: drinking among 11–15-year-old boys and girls doubled between 1990 and 2007;
- England and Wales came nearly top of the league in terms of drunkenness in early adolescence.

Case Study 7.1 illustrates how heavy drinking can lead to a high risk of casual sexual relationships in contexts where, for young women in particular, there is a loss of self-control and increased vulnerability.

CASE STUDY 7.1

Drink-related sexual relationships (adapted from Aldridge *et al.*, 2011: 79–81)

The researchers followed up a cohort of 14-year-olds until they were 18 years in order to study their drinking and use of recreational drugs. Here, one participant, Karen, describes the particular risks for young women that arise from intoxication.

> You know when you're out and that and you're bladdered. And you think, 'Oh that person's gorgeous', and then you come home and you don't remember a thing. And then when you're out the next week people say, 'That's the fella you got off with.' And you're just like, 'Oh I never.' That's happened a few times . . .

The interviews with young women also revealed that they had consulted their doctors about health problems related directly or indirectly to their drinking, including kidney problems, feeling generally 'run down' and blood poisoning. These young drinkers reported that they had to balance the negative effects of drinking with the positive, social benefits. They also indicated that, through a process of trial and error, they came to gauge their own limits and learned when it was time to stop. The researchers found that a proportion of the young people in their sample brought this 'cost-benefit assessment' with regard to alcohol consumption to their later experimentation with illegal drugs. This study provided evidence that many young people start drinking in their early teens and most drink regularly by their mid-teens. They make a transition from home-based drinking which is usually parent-supervised, to experimental drinking in public places, such as parks, through to drinking in licensed premises by the mid- to late teens. By the time they are 16, the majority report that they enjoy drinking; at the same time, around half of young drinkers report feeling unhappy afterwards, because of hangovers, headaches or vomiting.

Alcohol is central to the leisure activity of most young people throughout the adolescent years. Is it sufficient that they carry out their own risk assessment or should adults do more?

Alcohol consumption at a low age is linked to a range of poor outcomes, including antisocial behaviour and offending. A National Centre for Social Research survey (Institute of Alcohol Studies, 2009) found that in England, of 11–15-year-olds who had drunk in the past 4 weeks, 8% of boys and 7% of girls reported getting into trouble with the police after drinking. The prevalence of violent offending was higher among those who drank alcohol at least once a week (39%) in comparison with those who had not drunk alcohol in the past 12 months (11%). Although recent legislation aims to tackle under-age drinking in public spaces, many young people continue to misuse alcohol regularly in town centres, local streets and in parks. Many of these young people will have regular contact with crime reduction agencies but are only infrequently offered harm reduction interventions (Alcohol Concern, 2010). The risks for young people drinking unsupervised in open spaces are considerable, and include risk of overdose, violent attack or sexual assault (ibid.). For those young people who do enter the criminal justice system, youth offending teams have made good progress in recognizing, identifying and meeting alcohol-related needs in young people (Currie, 2010).

As is the case with alcohol, for many young people taking drugs is associated with social life among friends. The drugs most associated with early adolescence include amphetamines, amyl nitrate and solvents. Solvent abuse is the deliberate inhalation of household products, such as lighter gas refills, aerosols, deodorants and air fresheners, tins or tubes of glue, some paints and paint thinners, in order to feel intoxicated. Beinart *et al.* (2002) found that 7% of boys and 6% of girls in Year 7 (age 11–12) reported that they had sniffed solvents at least once. These percentages increased to 9% of males and 11% of females in Year 10, with a decrease in Year 11. The drug most commonly used by young people is cannabis. Currie *et al.* (2008) found that 25–35% of 15-year-olds in Europe reported having taken cannabis at least once in the past year. By contrast, no more than 5% report taking heroin or cocaine.

Pupils who have been excluded from school have consistently higher rates of alcohol use and drug-taking than non-excluded peers. By the time of adolescence, excluded children are more likely to drink regularly than non-excluded peers, with 46% reporting that they drink alcohol at least once a week compared with 26% of school children (Youth Justice Board, 2004). Excluded young people who have tried cannabis report a significantly higher level of usage on a weekly basis than their peers in school. Forty-five per cent of cannabis users have used the drug in the last month, with 38% having used it in the past week.

Health outcomes for alcohol, drugs and substance misuse

The link between heavy drinking and health is complex (Smith & Curran, 2010). Health risk factors include alcohol or drug dependence in later life, liver disease, high blood pressure, heart disease and oral and upper digestive cancers. There is a strong relationship between heavy drinking and admission to Accident and Emergency departments due to alcohol overdoses, accidents and involvement in violence. Alcohol dependency is also related to mental health difficulties. Young people who engage in heavy drinking are also significantly more likely to engage in unprotected sex.

On the basis of a number of studies of under-age drinking, Smith and Curran (ibid.: 8) report the following adverse effects on children and young people:

● Physiological factors resulting from a typically lower body mass and less effective metabolism of alcohol;
● Neurological factors due to changes in the brain that occur in young people after drinking alcohol;
● Cognitive factors, such as impaired judgement, which lead to a greater likelihood of accidents;
● Social factors which lead to intoxication and risk-taking behaviour.

The use of drugs presents a significant health hazard for young people, especially in circumstances where there is excessive use or where young people move on to hard drugs, such as cocaine and heroin. The risks from solvent abuse are also severe, causing nausea, vomiting, blackouts and heart problems that can be fatal. Long-term abuse of glue can cause damage to the brain, liver and kidneys (Field-Smith *et al.*, 2002) with longer-term outcomes that may persist into adulthood. Tate *et al.* (2008) found that **co-morbidity** – the presence of more than one major health disorder in an individual – led to a heightened risk of relapse for individuals with a combination of major depressive disorder and alcohol or substance dependence. This made treatment needs much more complex and could act against positive outcomes.

Interventions to prevent and treat alcohol, drugs and substance abuse

There is a strong case for schools to intervene early with educational programmes designed to prevent the harmful effects of alcohol, drugs and solvents. Approaches should be non-judgemental, use experiential learning methods and, if possible, involve parents/carers and members of the local community. Organizations, such as Alcohol Concern, provide a range of guides on school policy and practice and recommend such aspects as:

● The inclusion of alcohol and drug issues in the curriculum;
● The clarification of the use of alcohol on school trips;
● Addressing residential and social occasions with regard to alcohol;
● Addressing the drinking behaviour of school staff.

There has been considerable progress in the treatment of young people who use drugs. In the period from 2005 to 2010, the number of under-18s using cocaine, heroin, ecstasy and crack fell steadily, as reflected in the drop in the number of teenagers accessing services for help with drug problems. For example, at the time of writing, rates of accessing services for cocaine use dropped by 43% in the past two years and for ecstasy by 79% (National Treatment Agency for Substance Misuse, 2010). The number of under-18s completing treatment successfully more than doubled to 10,160 between 2005 and 2010. Most young people accessing services for help with dependence on cocaine, heroin, ecstasy and crack have not been taking drugs for long, but they are more likely to be heavy users, with ongoing physical, psychological and behavioural difficulties.

The majority of young people accessing services in 2009–2010 received counselling and behavioural therapies to address the underlying issues as well as the consequences of the substance misuse. They also received help with such outcomes as exclusion from school, breakdown of families, poor school attendance and health problems.

Recent innovative interventions that have been developed for adults offer some promise if they are adapted for young people. One example is the FRAMES Programme which takes the form of brief, instructive information on risks from alcohol, one-to-one sessions and motivational interviewing (see Box 7.1).

Box 7.1

FRAMES: an intervention (reported in Smith & Curran, 2010)

Brief interventions like FRAMES target people who have not necessarily acknowledged that they have an alcohol or drugs problem. A major advantage of this kind of brief intervention is that, after appropriate training, it can be delivered by non-specialists, so avoiding the stigma of attending a clinic. Additionally, this method builds on existing relationships that exist with adults, whether in school or in the community.

- Feedback is provided on the individual's risk for alcohol problems;
- Responsibility is taken by the target person for their own process of change;
- Advice is given on reduction of alcohol consumption and specific direction for change;
- A Menu provides a range of options for facilitating change;
- Empathy on the part of the facilitator demonstrates a warm, reflective and understanding approach;
- Self-efficacy encourages optimism about the potential for change.

Although it has been shown to be successful with adults, its effectiveness with children and young people is less clear-cut and further evaluation research is urgently needed. Of particular importance is the need to evaluate its effectiveness with potentially vulnerable groups, such as looked-after children or children with lower levels of literacy.

Discussion question

How could you adapt FRAMES to meet the needs of a younger age group? Design an effective poster. Plan an interactive DVD. Design a workshop to demonstrate the hazards of taking drugs or alcohol unsupervised in public spaces.

CASE STUDY 7.2

How 11-year-old Jason became dependent on alcohol

Jason started drinking when he was 11 years old. His parents had just split up and he found that drinking helped him not to feel so upset. He spent weekends at his Dad's house where there was plenty of alcohol and his Dad did not notice when Jason poured himself a glass or two from whatever bottle happened to be open. By the time he was 13, his consumption of alcohol increased from weekends only to almost every day. He started stealing from his Mum's purse so that he could buy his own alcohol from older boys who could pass for 18 at the off-licence. When she caught him stealing he began shoplifting and stealing from people in the community. Over time, it became harder for him to get up in the morning to go to school. He was irritable and lacked concentration.

Discussion question

What action might be taken to help Jason?

An example from one hospital Emergency Department (ED) illustrates the impact that intervention can have. In response to the needs of under-16s like Jason, Alder Hey Children's Hospital, Liverpool, has introduced a coding system to facilitate consistent intervention for children and young people who present at the ED with alcohol-related conditions. Each young person is screened, given an information pack and offered a follow-up appointment at the clinic within a week. At the clinic, qualified nurses, trained in motivational interviewing, deliver harm-reduction information (see Box 7.1). Since this brief intervention method was introduced, alcohol-related attendance at the ED has fallen from 210 attendances in 2005 to 64 attendances in 2009.

In the next section, we turn to another aspect of young people's lives – their eating behaviour – and the risks that this can pose for their health.

Obesity

The nature and incidence of obesity

Obesity is one of the most common medical problems affecting children and adolescents in Western and developing countries. The incidence of overweight and obesity is expected to rise and so presents society with a medical challenge for the future. There are a number of factors that cause children to become overweight. The most common causes are genetic factors, lack of physical activity and unhealthy eating, or a combination of these three. Very rarely, overweight is caused by a medical condition, such as a hormonal problem. Weight difficulties often run in families but not all children from families with a history of obesity will become overweight. Family eating habits and levels of activity play an important role here. A child's diet and level of physical activity significantly influence whether the child becomes overweight or not. Furthermore, to put the issue in its historical context, children in today's society, in comparison with children in the past, spend substantially more time doing sedentary activities such as sitting at the computer or watching television.

Definition

Obesity in childhood and adolescence can be broadly defined as excessive weight in relation to age or height. Some professionals consider a child to be obese if his/her body weight is at least 20% higher than a healthy weight for a child of that height, or if the child's body fat percentage is above 25% (for boys) or 32% (for girls). But what is meant by 'healthy weight'?

The most common measure of adult weight status is the **Body Mass Index** (**BMI**) which is weight in kilograms divided by the square of height in metres. The BMI thresholds are derived from European populations to correspond to risk thresholds for a range of chronic diseases. Adults are classified as overweight if their BMI is 25.0–29.9 kg/m^2 and obese if their BMI is 30 kg/m^2 and above.

However, the BMI is less appropriate for the measurement of children since fatness and BMI vary with age, ethnicity and gender (National Obesity Observatory (NOO), 2009). According to the NOO, the most commonly used reference charts for children in the UK are the British 1990 growth reference (UK90), using growth charts based on the UK population, and the International Obesity Task Force growth reference (IOTF), using growth charts based on pooled data from a range of countries and ethnicities – Brazil, the UK, the Netherlands, the USA, Singapore and Hong Kong. Using the UK90 growth reference to determine a child's BMI status, depending on age and gender, those whose BMI is between the 85th and less than the 95th centile are classified as *overweight*; those at or above the 95th centile are classified as *obese*.

Prevalence

The National Child Measurement Programme (NCMP) (2011, for data collection results from 2009/2010) annually records the height and weight measurements of children in Reception class (aged 4–5 years) and Year 6 (aged 10–11 years) attending state primary schools in England. According to the NCMP, the incidence of obesity in children is increasing. Here are some of the key findings reported in the NCMP report on the 2009/2010 school year:

- In Reception, 23.1% of children were overweight or obese. In Year 6, this rate was one in three (33.4%).
- The percentage of obese children in Year 6 (18.7%) was nearly double that of Reception (9.8%), whilst the percentage of overweight children was higher in Year 6 (14.6%) than in Reception (13.3%).
- The overall prevalence of underweight children was higher in Year 6 (1.3%) than in Reception (0.9%). In Reception, more boys were underweight than girls (1.1% and 0.7% respectively); whereas in Year 6, more girls were underweight than boys (1.5% and 1.1% respectively).

● Obesity prevalence varied by Strategic Health Authority (SHA) ranging from 8.4% in South East Coast SHA to 11.6% in London SHA for Reception, and from 16.1% in South West SHA to 21.8% in London SHA for Year 6.

The extent of child obesity varies substantially among different ethnic groups, with obesity prevalence usually lower in children of White British ethnicity (see Figures 7.1 and 7.2).

In 2009, an expert group investigated the representativeness of childhood obesity definitions, evidence for ethnic differences in body composition in UK children and the extent of mis-classification of obesity by current BMI thresholds (Viner *et al.*, 2010). They found that, using IOTF definitions, very few children were misclassified and the extent of misclassification was similar among S. Asian and White British young people. They concluded that the IOTF definitions of obesity remained the most appropriate for use in the UK. In other words, they recommended a single international BMI obesity threshold rather than ethnic-specific definitions for child obesity. They predicted that differences between ethnic groups may reduce with generations born in the UK. They also indicated that further research is needed on the relationship between body shape, fat mass, metabolic markers and ethnicity in children and adolescents.

With regard to overweight and obesity in different ethnic groups, the NCMP data (2011, for data collection results from 2009/2010) indicated the following (NOO, 2011: 11):

● Obesity prevalence was significantly higher than the national average for children in both school years in the ethnic groups: Asian or Asian British, 'Any Other' Ethnic Group, Black or Black British and 'Mixed'.

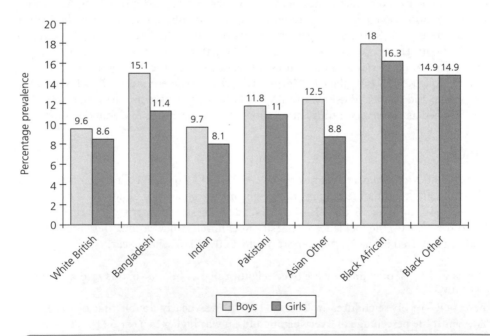

Figure 7.1 Percentage prevalence of obesity among 4–5-year-olds by ethnic group and gender.

Source: National Child Measurement Programme, 2009/2010.

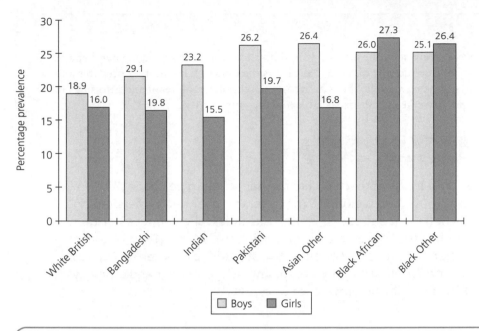

Figure 7.2 Percentage prevalence of obesity among 10–11-year-olds by ethnic group and gender.

Source: National Child Measurement Programme, 2009/2010.

- In Reception classes, obesity prevalence was especially high for both boys and girls from Black African and Black Other ethnic groups and boys from the Bangladeshi ethnic group.
- For girls in Year 6, the pattern was broadly similar to that observed for girls in Reception.
- For boys in Year 6, all ethnic groups reported significantly higher prevalence of obesity than the White British ethnic group, with boys of Bangladeshi ethnicity having the highest prevalence.
- The prevalence of obesity in some Asian groups was as high as, or higher than, that for the Black African and Black Other ethnic groups.

CASE STUDY 7.3

Should BMI thresholds be adapted for certain ethnic groups?

Fifteen-year-old Michelle, an active, confident teenager of African-Caribbean heritage, is overweight according to the BMI charts. Her form teacher is concerned about her health and would like her to consider changing her diet and lifestyle. But Michelle disagrees. She loves the food that her mother prepares and enjoys cooking as well. She is active in the school netball team and also sings in a band at weekends. She is sociable and has lots of friends.

Discussion questions

Should the form teacher take further action to persuade Michelle to control her weight? What are the chances of persuading Michelle that she faces health risks unless she changes her diet and lifestyle? Based on existing evidence, who is right: Michelle or her form teacher? Look at the statistics presented in Figures 7.1 and 7.2. How might you explain the age, gender and ethnicity differences in the prevalence of obesity?

Health and well-being outcomes

Being overweight has a number of psychological and health outcomes for children. Obese children are more likely to become overweight as adults, with an increased risk of heart disease, diabetes and stroke in adult life. Overweight children frequently experience social isolation and, as a consequence, develop poor self-esteem, stress and sadness. Obesity in adolescence may result in depression (Calamaro & Waite, 2009) which can continue through to adulthood (Doak *et al.*, 2006).

However, these outcomes need to be considered in their social context. Perceptions of weight and body image vary in different cultures and between generations. Not all cultures share the Western preference for leanness. In some cultures, being fat is a sign of wealth and success in life, so is highly valued. Cultural valuation of weight and shape can have a significant influence on the child's self-perception and emotional well-being. For example, Viner *et al.* (2010), in their study of East London adolescents, found that, for girls, obesity was associated with higher self-esteem among Black-African groups but with lower self-esteem among Bangladeshi groups. Among boys, obesity had a negative impact on self-esteem for those from both White and Bangladeshi groups.

See also Box 7.2 for a summary of risk factors for rapid weight gain in pre-schoolers. Here Griffiths *et al.* (2010) investigate factors, during pregnancy and in the early years of a child's life, that might contribute to the risk of becoming overweight or obese. In their discussion, they recommend that health education programmes should begin before and during pregnancy. They particularly target behaviours that are potentially under the control of the adults that care for the child, such as smoking and diet.

Box 7.2

Risk factors for rapid weight gain in pre-school children: findings from a UK-wide prospective study (Griffiths *et al.*, 2010)

This study as part of the nationally representative Millenium Cohort Study examined risk factors for weight gain in a sample of 11,653 young children aged between 3 and 5 years whose weight gain scores were calculated between the ages of 3 and 5 years. Children in the top quarter of this distribution were classified as gaining weight rapidly. A total of 26 biological and early-life, social, psychological, behavioural and environmental risk factors were examined.

The results indicated that 88% of obese 5-year-olds had experienced rapid weight gain since 3 years of age. Six biological and early-life factors and two social factors were found to be significantly associated with this growth pattern. The children who were more likely to gain weight rapidly:

- Had a higher BMI at age 3;
- Were of Bangladeshi or Black ethnicity;
- Had mothers who were overweight or had been overweight before pregnancy;
- Had fathers who were overweight;
- Had mothers who smoked during pregnancy;
- Had parents who smoked in the same room;
- Were only children in a predominantly adult household.

The researchers conclude that factors operating during pregnancy and early life increase the risk of rapid weight gain in young children.

Discussion question

What action might educators and healthcare professionals take?

Prevention and treatment of overweight and obesity

The UK government has identified obesity as a priority and has set targets to halt its rise year by year. As a result, there has been considerable action on the development of policies to address the issue (DH, 2004; Department of Health/Department of Education, 2009; Scottish Government, 2008). The National Institute for Health and Clinical Excellence (NICE) (2004, 2009b) has published guidelines for good practice in the community, in early-years settings, in schools and workplaces, as well as self-help recommendations. In 2008, the government established the Cross-Government Obesity Unit jointly led by the Department of Health and the Department of Education. This section describes a number of initiatives to reverse childhood obesity by tackling the social, psychological and physical environment of the child. There are a number of interventions that have been shown to reduce overweight in childhood and adolescence (adapted from NOO, 2011):

- In infancy, breastfeeding and delaying the introduction of solids can help prevent obesity;
- In early childhood, children's weight can be controlled by giving them healthy food and by discouraging consumption of high-fat snacks and sugary sweets in between meals;
- Children need to be encouraged to take lots of exercise;
- Parents can also limit sedentary activities, such as watching television and DVDs, surfing the internet and playing computer games;
- School-age children can be taught to select healthy, nutritious foods and to develop good exercise habits.

Parents need to be supportive in helping a child to lose weight by talking the issue through carefully and tactfully with their child. Whatever the intervention, parents/carers need to ensure that their child continues to feel good about him/herself. Doutre and Mansfield (2010) point out the dearth of studies that actually consult with children on the issue of overweight. They interviewed a small sample of 3 girls and 5 boys in Year 5 to elicit their views and found that the children displayed ambivalence in their attitudes towards overweight peers. On the one hand, participants in the study showed empathy and understanding of the difficulties that obese children face (ibid.: 17):

> Fat ain't a big deal, just coz you're fat it ain't the end of the world.

On the other hand, they stated that they did not want to be like obese children and were very aware of the barriers to quality of life that being overweight presents (ibid.: 19):

> Well the sad part is that you won't win a lot of races, coz the weight will be pulling you down.

The participants in this study recognized the risks of stigmatization and victimization as well as the likelihood of developing low self-esteem. They stated that being overweight was the result of unhealthy eating and sedentary lifestyles. With regard to intervention, the participants viewed obese children as having choices in their own destiny. Their suggested solutions indicated that they understood the importance of schools, families and professionals in helping individuals to change their lifestyle.

The evidence suggests that interventions to help obese children need to be linked to inclusion aspects of school policy. For example, schools could create safe places for overweight children to exercise without fear of ridicule and bullying. Peers might be encouraged to include overweight children in social activities by joining them in the activities of their choice. Hurtful, negative remarks could be challenged and replaced with supportive relationships, with the help of classmates and peer supporters in the school.

It is important that healthcare and educational professionals take account of the child's social and family context in order to understand the reasons that underlie a child's weight gain. It may also be essential to provide professional guidance in changing the eating and activity patterns of the family as a whole, rather than singling out the individual child.

Eating difficulties following a bereavement

Janice is 4 years old. She lives with her mum, Anne, and older sister, Jackie. Janice's father died suddenly a year ago. Janice's BMI is just above the 85th centile on the UK90 growth reference scale. Anne has asked for help from her GP, Dr Barnes, in managing Janice's weight. She has brought photographs of Janice at different ages to show that as a baby and toddler her weight appeared to be 'normal'. The family remains devastated by their loss. Anne admits that she did not cope well immediately after the death. One outcome was that she stopped cooking and instead relied on takeaways and convenience food which the family would eat as they watched television. Jackie is a very active, sociable child who loves sports and dancing; her weight has remained typical for her age. By contrast, Janice is 'clingy'. Anne has tried to enrol her at the local pre-school playgroup but Janice cries hysterically when Anne attempts to leave. She has few interests other than computer games and watching TV. Anne admits that Janice's food preferences are not very healthy but she does not like to refuse to allow her snacks as Janice gets so easily upset. After sensitive questioning Dr Barnes decides to refer Anne to Cruse for bereavement counselling. She also refers Anne and Janice to Active Families, a service that provides activities for parents and children together, such as hula hoop, trampolining, swimming, yoga, as well as opportunities to learn about healthy eating for the whole family.

Discussion questions

Dr Barnes has recommended therapeutic support for this mother as well as the opportunity for parent and child to be involved together in play activities and healthy eating education. Are there further interventions that would be helpful in addressing Janice's overweight? Are there other issues of concern in this family? What are the chances of success with this family?

Case Study 7.4 indicates that there may be emotional factors that affect weight, for example, following a significant loss or bereavement in the child's life. The child may be experiencing fears and anxieties about an aspect of family or school relationships. It is especially important not to make the parents or the child feel guilty, while, at the same time, stressing that the family has a key role to play in preventing further inappropriate weight gain.

Professionals need to be sensitive in the ways in which they approach discussion if they are to be successful in persuading the parents to accept help. They need to provide appealing opportunities for the child to be physically active, to develop an intrinsic motivation to make lifestyle changes and to avoid unhealthy preoccupation with weight.

In Case Study 7.4, the mother sought out professional help but this is not always the case. Where the parents or carers are not interested in support, or appear defensive, the professional should ensure that there are opportunities for the family to return for help when they are ready, or if the child is referred. There should also be awareness of the fact that some families live in 'obesogenic environments', such as areas of poverty, disadvantage and danger (O'Dea, 2005: 264). Families who live in such environments may lack facilities where children can play safely outside and may lack easy access to healthy food (see Case Study 7.5). Interventions could address these wider issues by helping to create sports and exercise facilities, better public transport and healthy food choices for children.

CASE STUDY 7.5

How can we safeguard a child when the parents/carers are reluctant to accept help?

Nine-year-old James is on the borderline of being classified as obese. He says that he is very unhappy as he has no friends and the other children laugh at him because of his size. He hates sports because no one ever chooses him to be in their team so, if possible, he avoids such activities. Recently he went to the school nurse complaining of breathlessness and dizziness. He told the nurse that the walk to school was making him very tired. The school nurse has invited his mum, Tracy, to come in to see her but Tracy is unenthusiastic and listless during the interview. Really, she says, there is very little that she can do to change James's weight. She claims that his condition is genetic since everyone in her family is 'big'. In any case, she reports, James strongly dislikes fruit and vegetables so it would be a waste of time to change his eating patterns. Also, he gets bullied in the local park so she doesn't let him go out to play. She herself is overweight and states firmly that she has no problems with it. The school nurse has indicated that, following a thorough assessment, Tracy and James could be referred to the free weight-management programme run by the School Nursing Service. This 24-session programme includes 1-to-1 consultations, measurements and goal-setting, physical activity and healthy eating activities. Very reluctantly Tracy agrees to attend.

Discussion questions

What are the chances of success with this family? How might the school nurse support James and Tracy? What happens if Tracy drops out of the weight-management programme?

Treatment

Treatment of childhood obesity should only occur with appropriate medical supervision and following a thorough clinical assessment. This ensures that children are assessed for risk factors and other related conditions. Treatment of obesity in children and adolescents requires not only diet and exercise but measures to address wider social and emotional issues such as self-esteem and social confidence. O'Dea (ibid.) argues strongly for the need to ensure that interventions do not cause the young person further harm, since health education messages about weight control can actually make young people feel worse about themselves and their bodies. Overemphasis on dieting, for example, can inadvertently lead to an upsurge in eating disorders. Media campaigns can often portray overweight children in a negative way as 'failures' or as individuals who lack self-control, so reinforcing self-blame, guilt, shame and hopelessness. Health and education professionals must ensure that their interventions do not unintentionally create anxiety around body image among the very population that they are trying to help, leading to potentially dangerous behaviours, such as starvation, vomiting, laxative abuse, slimming pill usage and cigarette smoking to suppress appetite (ibid.).

Some nutritionists (e.g., Bacon *et al.*, 2005) propose an emphasis on health improvement rather than on weight loss. The Health at Every Size (Bacon, 2008) movement recommends that a focus on a broad range of physical, psychological, social and spiritual dimensions in a child's life is more likely to have positive outcomes than simply dealing with weight alone. Health at Every Size encourages people to:

- Accept and respect the natural diversity of body sizes and shapes;
- Eat in a flexible way that values pleasure and honours internal cues of hunger, satiety and appetite;
- Find joy in moving one's body and becoming more physically vital.

Perspectives like these may increase the self-esteem of obese children and adolescents and encourage them to undertake more physical activity. They may also change prejudices against children whose size and weight are atypical. Dealing with the bullying and teasing that such children experience (Gracey *et al.*, 1996) may also help to enable healthy behaviours (see Box 7.3 for a summary of successful interventions).

Box 7.3

Effectiveness of interventions to reduce obesity in childhood and adolescence (based on Doak *et al.*, 2006)

On the basis of a systematic review of 25 school-based interventions focused on diet or activity-related behaviours, Doak *et al.* (ibid.) found that 17 of the 25 (68%) interventions were effective, based on a statistically significant reduction in BMI or skin-fold measurements for the intervention group. Four interventions were effective for both BMI and skin-fold reduction. Of these, two targeted reductions in television viewing and two targeted direct physical activity combined with nutrition education. The authors make the following recommendations:

- Future interventions should take body composition measures such as skin folds as well as height and weight in order to make more accurate assessments of body changes;
- More attention should be made by programme organizers to improving participation rates;
- There should be more awareness of the difficulty in targeting diverse groups, such as those that exist in large schools;
- Health promotion messages should be tailored appropriately according to ethnicity, gender and age;
- Interventions should directly alter the physical or social environment of the target group, for example, by altering menus in the school canteen or improving sports and exercise facilities in the school;
- More attention should be paid to sustainability of the changes over time by, for example, incorporating the intervention into the school curriculum;
- The impact of the intervention should be reported on the whole-school population, not only on children who are overweight or obese;
- Researchers should report on adverse outcomes, such as an increase in the incidence of underweight in the school population, or the stigmatization of obese children, or an increase in the potential for eating disorders.

There are many pressures on young people and their families with regard to size and weight. On the one hand, there is an increase in the incidence of overweight and obese children and, on the other hand, the media put great pressure on people to be thin and to be preoccupied with the shape and size of their bodies. As a result, some young people are very dissatisfied with their bodies and try to control their weight, shape and size through dieting, with potentially dangerous consequences, as indicated in the next section.

Eating disorders

The nature and incidence of eating disorders

During puberty, girls typically experience an increase in the amount of bodily fat while boys experience a decrease. Adapting to these changes can be very challenging for young people. This is a time when dissatisfaction with the body increases, with girls expressing significantly more dissatisfaction with their bodies than boys (Paxton & Heinicke, 2008), especially with regard to fat on hips, buttocks, stomach and thighs. Adolescent boys worry about their weight but are more likely to strive to be muscular rather than thin. One outcome is that some young people increasingly experience a discrepancy between their own bodies and the ideal bodies that are promoted through the media and the culture of celebrities (Keel *et al.*, 2007; Paxton & Heinicke, 2008). Dieting is a risk factor for eating disorders during adolescence with

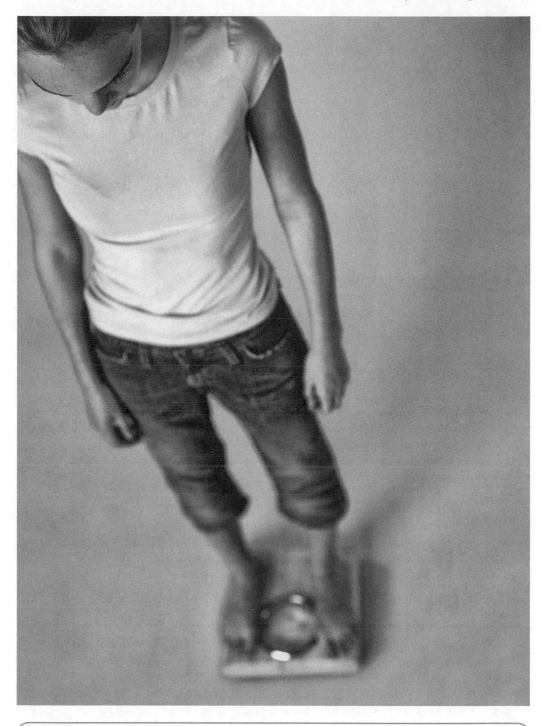

Ian Boddy/Getty images

outcomes that include depression, anxiety and lower self-esteem. In particular, when dieting is accompanied with negative feelings about the self, this can lead to more severe eating disorders. Eating disorders alter the person's cognitive ability, judgement and emotional stability.

There are two major types of eating disorder – **anorexia nervosa** and **bulimia nervosa**. Each is likely to present initially as a physical disorder involving extreme dietary restriction and various forms of extreme weight-control behaviour, such as self-induced vomiting, obsessive exercising or laxative misuse. Common features include fear of being fat, self-evaluation based on shape and weight, extensive efforts to control weight, relationship difficulties and increasing withdrawal from social life. A person can show both anorexic and bulimic eating patterns at different times.

Anorexia nervosa is characterized by the following:

- Refusal to maintain body weight at or above a minimally normal weight for age and height;
- Intense fear of becoming fat, even when underweight;
- Distorted body image;
- Denial of the seriousness of current low body weight;
- Food avoidance.

A person with bulimia nervosa alternates between eating very little and then having binges when they eat too much. The characteristics of bulimia nervosa include:

- An overwhelming urge to overeat, leading to binges; a sense of not being able to control eating during the episode;
- Recurrent compensatory behaviour, such as self-induced vomiting, laxative abuse, excessive fasting or exercise;
- The binge eating and compensatory behaviour both occur, on average, at least twice a week for three months;
- Self-evaluation is unduly influenced by body shape and weight;
- A morbid fear of becoming fat.

Eating disorders not otherwise specified (EDNOS): in addition, there are some young people who do not meet all of the criteria for anorexia nervosa or bulimia nervosa but who demonstrate atypical eating patterns. For example, they may show all the signs of anorexia nervosa but still manage to maintain a normal weight, or they may binge by chewing and spitting out rather than swallowing. These people are classified as having an eating disorder not otherwise specified (EDNOS).

Incidence

In the UK, anorexia nervosa affects around 1 in 100 women aged between 15 and 30 years. Usually this illness begins in adolescence but in rare cases it begins in childhood. The illness affects approximately 1 in 150 15-year-old females and 1 in 1,000 15-year-old males. Recently, however, there has been a worrying increase in eating disorders among boys and young men. Anorexia nervosa may start following a period of dieting in response to being called fat or, less frequently, following a viral infection, but often there are deeper emotional issues. For example, a history of sexual abuse is reported in 3 out of 10 people with anorexia nervosa. Risk factors include: relationship difficulties in the family; bereavement or loss of a significant person; low self-esteem; high aspirations to achieve; being bullied about weight; severe stresses in life; a change of school; use of recreational drugs; the onset of depression. Young people with anorexia nervosa will often hide their eating difficulties. They spend a great deal of time feeling anxious about food, exercise, body size and appearance. It has a high morbidity and mortality rate and can persist for many years.

Bulimia nervosa usually begins during adolescence. The prevalence is 1–3% in girls and 0.1–0.3% in boys. The main risk factors for bulimia include: family history of obesity; personal history of obesity; parental history of depression; personal history of depression; being teased about weight or shape; negative feelings about the self; parental alcoholism.

Outcomes for eating disorders

Eating disorders lead to a range of negative effects on the person including:

- Feeling very cold;
- Headaches;
- Changes in hair and skin;
- Tiredness;
- Stunting of growth;
- Loss of periods and fertility in girls;
- Anxiety and depression;
- Poor concentration;
- Withdrawal from friends and family.

Anorexia nervosa has a less favourable outcome with regard to both remission and mortality than bulimia nervosa (Keel & Brown, 2010). Mortality figures range from 1–8% of cases with anorexia nervosa and 0–2% of cases with bulimia nervosa. Even after recovering, many cases still suffer from psychological problems for several years.

Treatment for eating disorders

Young people with an eating disorder are likely to be experiencing strong feelings of self-disgust, acute anxiety and depression. In this vulnerable state, they need to be treated with great care and sensitivity. It is essential to seek expert medical help. One-to-one counselling, such as **Cognitive Behavioural Therapy (CBT)**, can help the young person to understand the reasons that underlie their negative feelings about themselves. CBT in particular facilitates examination of the links between thoughts, feelings and behaviour so as to begin the process of eating regularly and in a healthy way. Participation in therapeutic groups that focus on anger management, problem-solving and assertiveness can also help young people to understand themselves and to embark on the process of change. Nursing staff and dieticians can provide guidance on healthy eating. Young people also benefit from programmes that enhance self-esteem and social skills. Case Study 7.6 describes some of the typical aspects of the disorder.

CASE STUDY 7.6

How Alicia overcame anorexia nervosa

When Alicia was 15, she and her friends all decided to go on a diet at the same time in order to drop a dress size. The girls were under a great deal of pressure at school to do well in their exams. To Alicia, dieting seemed to offer a way of controlling her anxiety about not being academic enough to please her parents, whose long-standing ambition was that she would win a place at Oxford, just as they had done themselves. Alicia had already had a setback when she was not shortlisted for a place at a famous ballet school. She was convinced that she had overheard one of the members of the interview panel say that she was 'too big to be a ballerina'. Alicia was known to be a perfectionist and the dieting regime presented her with a challenge. Most of the girls quickly lapsed from the diet as they felt so hungry all the time. But Alicia persisted and soon began to lose weight, as she had planned. It was initially very satisfying to see the effects of her disciplined approach to food. At first she weighed herself every morning but as the weeks went on she found herself impelled to go on the scales every time she went into the bathroom. She also became obsessed with the calories in every mouthful she ate. Whenever the scales indicated that she had gained a few pounds, she began to reduce her food intake further and to take laxatives to purge her body of food. Despite this, she still felt fat. Her friends began to comment on her weight loss but that made her very self-conscious so she stopped going out with them. In any case, she did not have the energy to go out much and started to feel ill and tired all the time. Her skin changed and her hair became lacklustre and brittle. She began to hate the way she looked.

Although she became good at hiding her dieting behaviour, eventually her mother noticed how often she made excuses not to eat. Her father became very angry and insisted that she finish her meals while he watched her. This only made the situation worse since she would then rush to the bathroom and make herself vomit. Mealtimes became tense occasions of anger, hurt and recrimination.

Eventually, her mother became so alarmed at what was happening that she persuaded Alicia to go to the GP who referred her to the local Child and Adolescent Mental Health Service (CAMHS) team, including a nurse, a psychiatrist, a psychologist and a family therapist.

The team offered a range of support services. Alicia received one-to-one CBT, she and her parents were offered a series of family therapy sessions, and she was given guidance on healthy eating and enjoyable exercise routines. The treatment took 5 months but at the end Alicia began to feel much better about herself and her body. Her parents had learned during family therapy not to put excessive pressure on her but to allow her to develop at her own pace. Alicia began to rebuild relationships with her peer group and to return to her original passion for a contemporary dance class where the teacher actively celebrated diversity in shape and appearance.

Chapter summary

Drugs and alcohol misuse: Taking drugs and alcohol is very prevalent among young people. There are increasing concerns about the health risks involved. There is a strong case for early intervention to provide young people with the relevant information. Approaches should be non-judgemental and should, where possible, involve families and the local community. A range of methods for treating addiction are discussed.

Overweight and obesity: Overweight and obesity are increasing as health concerns in childhood and adolescence. There are a number of factors that contribute to overweight and obesity. These include genetic factors, lack of physical activity, unhealthy eating patterns or a combination of all three. Western societies have also placed too much emphasis on slimness, so causing many young people to be dissatisfied with their body size, shape and weight. Some environments have an adverse effect on healthy eating, for example, areas of deprivation and poverty where access to sports may be limited and where the community may be a dangerous place. There has been some questioning of childhood obesity thresholds since they vary by ethnicity. A number of interventions have been proved to reduce overweight in childhood. These include: attention to healthy eating during pregnancy; encouraging children to be active and to avoid sedentary behaviours such as excessive TV viewing; promoting healthy eating at school.

Eating disorders: There are two major types of eating disorder: anorexia nervosa and bulimia nervosa. Young people with an eating disorder experience feelings of self-disgust, anxiety and depression. There are serious physical and psychological outcomes which need to be treated urgently and under expert medical supervision. There are a number of proven interventions that can help young people with an eating disorder. These include one-to-one counselling, therapeutic group work and sensitive and informative guidance on healthy eating. Schools also have an important part to play in heightening awareness about the importance of healthy eating.

> **Discussion points**
>
> ● Research has shown that BMI may not always be the best way to measure obesity; for example, for the same level of BMI, children of African ethnicity seem to carry less fat, which may lead to an overestimation of obesity among African groups. How can healthcare professionals balance the need to be respectful of cultural differences and the need to safeguard children's health?
>
> ● Some communities are reported to be 'obesogenic'. What can be done to support families who live in such circumstances?
>
> ● Some communities are plagued by excessive drinking on the part of young people in open spaces and local streets and town centres. Should the police enforce stronger sanctions or should more attention be paid to the social and emotional issues of the young people concerned?

Further reading

DrugScope provides a very useful free resource: McWhirter, J. & Mir, H. (eds) (2008) *The Essential Guide to Working with Young People about Drugs and Alcohol*, London: DrugScope. Aldridge, J., Measham, F. & Williams, L. (2011) *Illegal Leisure Revisited: Changing Patterns of Alcohol and Drug Use in Adolescents and Young Adults*, London: Routledge, updates the findings through to adulthood from a longitudinal study of a cohort of 14–18-year-olds that focused on their early drinking and regular use of recreational drugs.

The National Children's Bureau identifies positive ways of addressing obesity in childhood and adolescence in: Reilly, J. (2009) *Obesity in Childhood and Adolescence*, Highlight No. 250, London: National Children's Bureau. An ongoing systematic review of evidence on the effect of interventions to tackle obesity can be found in: Aicken, C., Arai, L. & Roberts, H. (2008) *Schemes to Promote Healthy Weight Amongst Obese and Overweight Children*, EPPI Centre, Institute of Education, University of London, Report No. 1607. For a psychological perspective, see: Cullen, K. (2011) 'Obesity in children', in J. A. Waumsley *et al.* (eds) (2011) *Obesity in the UK: A Psychological Perspective*, British Psychological Society Obesity Working Party, Leicester: BPS, www.bps.org.uk

Websites and resources

Fergus Currie reports on young people's misuse of alcohol in *Message in a Bottle*:
www.cqc.org.uk/_db/_documents/Inspecting_Youth_Offending_Thematic_-_Alcohol_Misuse_-

The Department of Health guidance on the consumption of alcohol by children and young people can be downloaded from:
http://www.dh.gov.uk/

The Institute of Alcohol Studies provides helpful information, factsheets and resources relating to problem drinking among youth on:
www.ias.org.uk/resources/factsheets/adolescents_problems.pdf

The National Obesity Observatory provides statistics and research findings on obesity and ethnicity in:
http://www.noo.org.uk/NOO_pub/briefing_papers

For a psychological perspective on obesity written for the British Psychological Society Obesity Working Party see K. Cullen's chapter 'Obesity in children', in J. A. Waumsley *et al.* (eds) (2011) *Obesity in the UK: A Psychological Perspective*:
www.bps.org.uk

Advice for parents about how to talk to their children about drugs can be found on:
www.talktofrank.com/

A website designed to help young people assess their own cannabis use is:
www.knowcannabis.org.uk

DrugScope provides a full range of information and resources on drug issues on:
www.drugscope.org.uk

as does Addaction on:
www.addaction.org.uk

Rethink provides information and discussion boards about cannabis and mental health:
www.rethink.org

and Mind provides general information about mental health issues on:
www.mind.org.uk

Alcohol Concern has a comprehensive website, including recent publications such as *Right Time, Right Place*, on alcohol-harm reduction strategies with children and young people:
http://www.alcoholconcern.org.uk/

Chapter 8

Safe and risky sexual behaviour

Map of the chapter

This chapter explores typical sexual development, as well as aspects of precocious, problematic and inappropriate sexual behaviours. It examines some of the common social and health risks arising from unprotected sex, including sexually transmitted diseases and unplanned pregnancy.

Sexual health

The nature of sexual health

> Sexual health is a state of physical, emotional, mental and social well-being related to sexuality; it is not merely the absence of disease, dysfunction or infirmity. Sexual health requires a positive and respectful approach to sexuality and sexual relationships, as well as the possibility of having pleasurable and safe sexual experiences, free of coercion, discrimination and violence. For sexual health to be attained and maintained, the sexual rights of all persons must be respected, protected and fulfilled.
>
> (World Health Organization, 2002)

Sexual exploration and play are a natural part of a child's development and help children to learn about their own bodies and also about the rules that govern behaviour in their particular culture. Children's sexual behaviour develops over time from infancy onwards. Children from an early age typically show curiosity about their own bodies, are interested in talking about sex and reproduction, and will often joke within the family or in the peer group about sexual matters. For infants and toddlers, sexual behaviour can take the form of bodily sensations, touching their own genitals and, in boys, experiencing erections. With the onset of puberty, young people experience changes in their bodies and become increasingly aware of sexual feelings and emotions.

Box 8.1

Typical sexual development and sexual play

- 1–5 years: babies and toddlers show curiosity about their own genitals; experience bodily sensations; touch and rub their own genitals.
- 5–7 years: children continue to be interested in body parts; demonstrate some sexual play; ask questions about sexual concepts; some girls show interest in using make-up and having their ears pierced.
- 8–9 years: children continue to show interest in sexual play, such as kissing and flirting; many have close girlfriends or boyfriends; children can express some understanding of love and relationships; these behaviours and questions continue developing into later childhood. By 9 years, some girls start menstruating.
- 10–12 years: children continue to be very aware of peer relationships; some experience sexual feelings; some children experience intense same-sex 'crushes'; touching of genitalia can evolve into masturbation/solo sex; not uncommon that boys and girls experiment with oral sex and, in some cases, penetrative sex. Boys often worry about penis size. They may have distorted views on what is 'normal' in terms of size and performance.
- 12–16 years: clearer patterns of sexual behaviour appear; onset of puberty; sexual organs develop for most by this age; menstruation happens for most girls; masturbation/solo sex is common, though more prevalent in boys; romance and intimacy integrate with sexual feelings and emotions; dating becomes more common; more sexual aspects to relationships, such as kissing and, for some, full sexual intercourse, including oral and anal sex. Some boys engage in solo sex on the internet and may post images to other boys and girls.

Currie *et al.* (2008) found that young people are becoming sexually active at an earlier age, with over 30% reporting having had sex by the age of 16; this trend has been rising since the 1960s. Young people wish to experiment and are less inhibited than in previous generations. The peer group can put pressure on young people to prove themselves sexually. For example, body-piercing and tattooing can demonstrate to peers that a young person has made the transition to manhood. The proof can be circulating intimate pictures of, for example, genital or belly button piercing, on the internet or by mobile phone. Young people are often unaware of the health risks involved in these practices. They will often rely more on blogs and informal chat with one another in order to seek clarification about sexual behaviour. Barter (2009) found in a survey of 1,353 young people aged 13–17 years that 88% reported some form of intimate sexual relationship. Research by Moore and Rosenthal (2006) indicates that young people are engaging in a wide range of sexual behaviours, including solo sex, anal and oral sex. At the age of 16, Black males are more likely to report that they are sexually active than are males from other ethnic groups, with Asian young people reporting the lowest rates at this age (Testa & Coleman, 2006). It is worth considering these findings when trying to understand the factors that influence the context and timing of adolescent sexual behaviour.

- Why are there differences between different ethnic minority groups in the extent to which they report being sexually active during adolescence?

Same-sex and opposite-sex relationships

Forming romantic relationships with peers is crucial for the development of young people's sexual and social identities. Involvement in romantic relationships gives young people an important opportunity to explore relationships with different kinds of partners in order to discover what they are looking for with regard to intimacy and commitment in the longer term. Concurrent sexual relationships are not uncommon in adolescence, to boost self-esteem and to experiment and 'practise' with different partners. Positive experiences of dating can be very beneficial for the young person's self-esteem and confidence. But sometimes there is confusion in the minds of young people as they may experience intense emotions about both same-sex and opposite-sex peers. For those youths who do not identify themselves as heterosexual (often referred to as sexual minorities) there are distinct difficulties, as they often face prejudice and discrimination from family, peers and others in their communities. There is evidence that many sexual-minority youths also engage in romantic relationships with opposite-sex partners, possibly to reduce the stigma and negative peer responses or simply in order to explore their evolving sexual identity (Bauermeister *et al.*, 2010).

CASE STUDY 8.1

'Am I gay?'A 12-year-old's letter to an agony aunt

I have always fancied boys, but lately I have been having feelings for girls, I don't know what's happening! Me and my best friend (who is also a girl) kissed before, but we didn't speak much of it, we both said we were feeling that way, but a few weeks later, she said she's passed that 'stage', but I don't think I have, is it just a stage? Please help!

Discussion questions

How can an adult reassure this girl that her feelings are very typical? How safe would it be for her to discuss her fears with friends or family?

Bauermeister *et al.* (ibid.) investigated the influence of same-sex and opposite-sex relationships on symptoms of depression, anxiety, internalized homophobia and self-esteem over time in a sample of 350 gay, lesbian or bisexual youths aged 15–19 in New York City. They found that the protective effects of same-sex relationships are different for young men and young women. A same-sex relationship is protective since it reduces internalized homophobia for girls, even after only one relationship. For young men, however, a same-sex relationship raises self-esteem but only if the relationship is long term. The researchers also found that it was beneficial for young people's self-esteem if they 'came out' to their friends. They recommend the value of creating supportive environments where young people can talk about their sexual identity. This may include being able to talk about experiences with same-sex and opposite-sex partners.

However, there are risks and benefits involved in coming out as gay, lesbian or bisexual. Young people in ethnic minority families, or those from families with very strong religious beliefs, for example, Muslim or evangelical Christian families, can experience great difficulty in coming out because of pressure from the community. Sexual-minority youth experience greater psychological distress than heterosexual youth and are highly likely to be bullied through verbal taunts, physical threats and physical violence (Rivers, 2011; Rivers & D'Augelli, 2001).

There are also risks for young people who have opposite-sex relationships. Barter *et al.* (2009) carried out a survey among 1,353 young people aged 13–17 years on their experiences of physical, emotional and sexual abuse and found it to be widespread. Having an older partner is a serious risk factor for girls. The statistics are disturbing. Barter *et al.* (ibid.) found that 25% of girls and 18% of boys who were 'in a relationship' reported that they had experienced some form of physical partner violence. One in 9 girls and 4% of boys reported severe violence. Seventy-five per cent of girls with partners who were at least two years older than them had experienced physical abuse; 80% had experienced emotional violence; 75% had experienced sexual violence. (See also Papadopoulos, 2010.)

There is growing evidence of pressure on adolescent girls to engage in sexual behaviour whether they feel ready or prepared for it or not. Teenage partner violence is also reported to be on the increase. Barter (2011) found that young people who reported some form of family violence towards themselves were more likely to have experienced an intimate relationship and more likely to experience one at an earlier age than young people with no history of domestic violence in their families. Young people who reported family violence were more likely to have experienced an intimate relationship at a younger age than young people with no history of domestic violence. Girls with a history of family violence were also more likely to have an older partner.

Barter (ibid.: 108) found that boys often reported disproportional violence in a dispute with their partner, as Case Study 8.2 indicates:

CASE STUDY 8.2

Partner violence (adapted from Barter & Berridge, 2011)

Interviewer: Did she hit you first?
Hardeep: Yes.

Interviewer: And were you shocked when it happened, or did you think she was going to do it?

Hardeep: I was a bit shocked . . . 'cos she didn't stop did she and you can't not hit a girl if she is attacking you . . . I think I let it happen again a few more times and then I hit her forehead and she got knocked out and we broke up.

In another part of the interview, Hardeep describes further incidents with other girlfriends where he justified his use of violence, so indicating that this was a pattern in his sexual relationships. For many teenage girls, the first experience of physical violence from a partner occurs when they refuse to have sexual intercourse (Barter, 2011).

Discussion question

How effective might school-based awareness-raising programmes be in preventing this type of violence?

The UK government has responded to the evidence on teenage partner violence by setting up the Violence Against Women and Girls (VAWG) Advisory Group which identified teenage relationship violence as a priority. Fortunately, there is some evidence that preventive programmes in schools can have an impact in heightening young people's awareness of dating violence and give them coping strategies for dealing with it should it occur. One example is the Healthy Relationships Programme which is delivered through a school's Personal, Social and Health Education (PSHE) curriculum. Evaluation of its impact on the young people immediately after the series of lessons, and one year later, indicated that most participants enjoyed taking part. With regard to changing attitudes, girls seemed to be more influenced than boys. However, generally the programme was successful in teaching the young people about individual rights to autonomy, privacy and freedom in relationships, as these quotations indicate (Stanley *et al.*, 2011: 220 and 226):

Both partners have an equal say. No one should make someone do what they don't want to. No one should get hurt. (Girl, aged 12–13 years)

To listen and look after my partner and try to understand her. (Boy, aged 12–13 years)

I would like to have it again – in Year 11 so I could keep it in mind – to learn it again in case I forgot. (Boy, aged 12–13 years)

These qualitative findings indicate that there is hope that professionals can deliver such programmes successfully. The study also indicates the importance of taking account of gender differences in the delivery and follow-up of such programmes.

Harmful sexual behaviours

In the light of current trends, it is difficult to be absolutely precise about the boundaries between healthy and unhealthy sexual development during childhood and adolescence. Furthermore, the ways in which sexual behaviours are defined as 'appropriate' or 'inappropriate' are culturally and historically influenced. The internet and films often 'normalize' violence within sexual relationships. Drugs and alcohol can also fuel violent and abusive sexual behaviour. This section explores sexual behaviours that are deemed to be harmful to the child/young person or to others in their social environment.

Hackett (2011) makes a useful distinction between sexual behaviours that are problematic and those that are abusive. **Sexually abusive behaviour** indicates sexual behaviours initiated by a child or young person where there is use of manipulation or force, or where the target is unable to give informed consent. **Sexually problematic behaviour** indicates sexual activity that may interfere with the child's development or increase that child's risk of rejection or victimization.

Precocious sexual behaviours in childhood become a cause for concern when they are excessively prominent in a child's life or when the behaviours intrude into the lives of other children. Examples of this would be when there is excessive sexual play, frequent incidence of rude, sexual comments, attempts at sexual activity with other children or actual sexual abuse of peers (Barnes, 2003). The majority of children who display such behaviours have been sexually abused or maltreated (Gray *et al.*, 1999). (See also Case Study 3.1.)

CASE STUDY 8.3

Paul's inappropriate sexual behaviour: a cry for help

Paul, aged 9, was referred to the school nurse following complaints from parents that he had been touching girls in his class in a sexual way. He was referred on to social services as the nurse quickly realized that there were serious family abuse issues in this case. Paul's parents had split up years ago and his father no longer played any part in his life. His mother, Tracy, had recently become involved with Mike who had moved into the family home, despite the fact that Paul disliked him and was quite afraid of him. Family life soon became very turbulent. Paul frequently experienced domestic violence and, on more than one occasion, had witnessed abusive sexual activity between his mum and her boyfriend. On occasion, when Mike was alone with Paul, he had touched his genitals. Paul became aroused and afterwards felt very ashamed. Mike said that this was their secret and Paul must not tell Tracy. His mum was now pregnant and Paul was desperately afraid that she would no longer be interested in him once the new baby arrived. Following intensive family support and counselling, Tracy developed a more nurturing approach to Paul and reassured him that she would still love him after the birth of the new baby. She was horrified to discover that Mike had been 'grooming' Paul. When she confronted him, Mike said that he

---

had just been teaching Paul the facts of life. Tracy made the decision to break off relations with Mike for the sake of her children. In this case, Paul's precocious sexual behaviour was a cry for help and expressed his deep insecurity about relationships within his family. With the creation of a more nurturing family environment, he no longer displayed inappropriate sexual behaviours.

Discussion questions

How understanding would Paul's school community be following his family's support and counselling? What are the chances that Paul will no longer feel the need to engage in inappropriate sexual activity?

Most pre-adolescents with sexual behaviour problems, like Paul, are vulnerable children who are trying to resolve feelings of anger, shame and confusion around sex and sexuality (Johnson & Doonan, 2005). Research findings indicate that, with appropriate therapeutic intervention and ongoing support, most can be helped and reintegrated back into their families and communities (Hackett, 2011).

In the case of adolescents with harmful sexual behaviour, the situation is more complex because of the diversity of behaviours (including the degree of force used, the levels of sexual arousal and the age and gender of the targeted victims) and the wider range of factors which underlie the behaviour. For example, adolescent abusers can be individuals with poor social skills and low self-esteem, who are rejected by their peers, and have difficulty in forming intimate relationships. They find their sexual gratification by seeking out much younger children. On the other hand, the adolescent abuser may be a person who is successful in attracting sexual partners but who has higher levels of non-sexual criminality, antisocial behaviour and violence, as well as aggression within sexual relationships. For those who are not in touch with their own anger, this can get in the way of good communication with sexual partners. The vast majority of adolescents with harmful sexual behaviours are male and the onset of puberty is a peak time for the development of such behaviours (Taylor, 2003).

By contrast, Matthews *et al.* (1997) found that young women who sexually abuse others had typically experienced chronic and extensive maltreatment in their childhood. Matthews and colleagues identified three distinct categories of female abuser:

- Those whose sexually abusive behaviour was an isolated incident, driven by curiosity, for example, while babysitting;
- Those whose sexually abusive behaviour was triggered by their own recent experience of sexual victimization;
- Those who had experienced high levels of abuse and neglect throughout their childhood. These young women were typically depressed, anxious and showing symptoms of post-traumatic stress disorder (PTSD).

The Teenage Pregnancy Common Assessment Framework Checklist (2010) identifies the following risk factors associated with harmful sexual behaviour:

High risk

- First sex under 16 years old and poor contraceptive use;
- Multiple sexual partners;
- Demonstrating or exposed to risky sexual behaviours;
- Vulnerable to sexual abuse and exploitation;
- Repeated access to emergency hormonal contraception.

Moderate risk

- Alcohol or drug use;
- Being in care or leaving care;
- Being a teenage parent;
- Poor levels of educational attainment or disengaged from school;
- Low self-esteem or poor emotional health;
- Involvement in youth offending;
- Poor family support/domestic violence;
- Growing up in an area of deprivation and poverty;
- Child protection concerns;
- Accessing abortion services;
- Being the child of a teenage parent.

In the light of these complex risk factors, intervention must target not only the harmful sexual behaviour but also the more general areas of need in the lives of these young people. The families of such young people are more likely to be troubled and dysfunctional, with a high likelihood that they feature domestic violence, or parental criminality, or a lack of sexual boundaries, or a history of sexual abuse within the family. This means that the parents themselves are in need of help and, as Hackett (2011) suggests, supporting parents is often a precursor to helping the family to face up to the impact that sexual abuse and neglect has on their children.

One widely used assessment framework is the Assessment, Intervention, Moving On Project (AIM) model (Print *et al.*, 2001) which focuses on the following domains:

- *Offence-specific factors*: the young person's offending history, the nature of the offence, previous history;
- *Developmental issues*: the young person's experience of abuse and neglect, the quality of their family life in the early years;
- *Family*: how well the family functions; family attitudes; sexual boundaries; parental competence;
- *Environment*: opportunities for future offending and the extent of support offered in the community.

This kind of model enables the practitioner to focus on risks and protective factors in the young person's environment in order to develop an appropriate form of intervention specific to the individual's particular needs and circumstances. The interventions that work best are those that are holistic and multi-modal. They must focus on the abusive sexual behaviour but they should also respond to broader developmental and social aspects in the young person's life. With appropriate diagnosis and treatment, a significant number of adolescents with harmful sexual behaviours do not reoffend (Hackett, 2011).

A new clinical trial is currently under way in the Brandon Centre for Counselling and Psychotherapy for Young People, a charitable organization, to evaluate the effectiveness of multi-systemic therapy (MST) to treat young people with problem sexual behaviour. MST therapists work with families in their homes and other community settings, meeting the families three or four times a week and being on-call around the clock, seven days a week. MST has been successful in the USA since in the majority of cases the young people do not reoffend.

Unprotected sexual activity

One outcome of increased sexual activity and, in particular, unsafe and risky sexual behaviours in young people has been the rise in sexually transmitted infections (STIs) such as Chlamydia and Human Papillomavirus (HPV) and HIV/AIDS, each of which has potentially serious long-term consequences. Young African-Caribbean men have higher rates of STIs. This may be due to peer-group pressure to prove masculinity and virility through unprotected sexual behaviour. The incidence of Chlamydia infection has doubled since 1998 (Coleman & Brooks, 2009). In a review of the health of people in England today, including sexual health, the Department of Health (2010) reports that, of all 15–24-year-olds diagnosed with an STI in the previous year, around 1 in 10 will become reinfected within a year. Clearly, this issue poses a major challenge to public health.

There are a number of reasons why young people engage in unprotected sexual activity. For younger adolescents, there may be practical reasons why they are unable to purchase condoms. They may also be embarrassed about discussing the question of contraception or be led to believe that using condoms is unmanly. They may be under the influence of alcohol or drugs and so not be in a rational frame of mind once sexual activity begins. Urban myths prevail

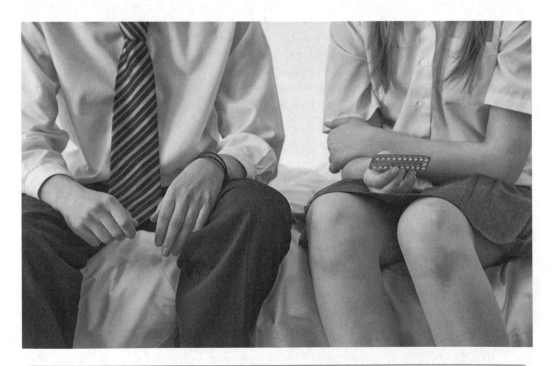

Getty images

among young people, for example, 'You don't become pregnant the first time you have sex', or 'You don't get pregnant if you have sex standing up.' There may be peer pressure to engage in sex. They may not understand that oral and anal sex does not necessarily protect a young woman from pregnancy.

Certain groups of young people are especially vulnerable to engaging in unprotected sex. These include: young women with low self-esteem, especially when involved with an older partner; young people from families where there is domestic violence or abuse; young people in areas of poverty and deprivation; young people who have been placed in care; young people who are at risk of being exploited; and young women from Muslim or evangelical Christian families who may experiment with oral and anal sex in order to protect their virginity. (See also the government review on the sexualization of young people (Papadopoulos, 2010).)

Teenage pregnancy

Not surprisingly, a further outcome of engaging in unprotected sex is unplanned pregnancy. The UK has one of the highest rates of teenage pregnancy in Europe. In the UK, the Department of Health/Department of Education (2009) made it a priority to reduce the number of teenage pregnancies, including those which end in a live birth and those that are terminated. In the UK, any sexually active young person under the age of 13 years must by law be referred to safeguarding agencies.

The Office for National Statistics (ONS) (2011b) identified a clear link between social deprivation and rates of teenage pregnancy, with young women from socially deprived areas more likely to become pregnant. The Department of Health/Department of Education (2009) also documents links between the age of the mother at the time of conception and poorer socio-economic outcomes for both mother and child. The chances of a young woman becoming pregnant before the age of 20 years are much greater for those who live in socially deprived areas. The most at-risk groups are: young people excluded from school; young people in care or leaving care; daughters of teenage mothers; young people involved in crime; some ethnic minority groups; vulnerable young people. Teenage pregnancy is also linked to a lack of knowledge about sex and relationships.

Borkowski et al. (2007) carried out a longitudinal study of a sample of 281 teenage mothers and their children, born in the late 1980s and early 1990s, across the first 14 years of their lives. They examined the risks but also identified factors of resilience in this cohort of young parents. With attrition, the sample reduced over time as follows: at 6 months, 25%; at 1 year, 8%. By the time the children were 14 years, the sample had reduced to 102 mothers. The young mothers experienced a number of social and emotional difficulties during pregnancy and were in general less well-prepared for parenting than adult women. At three, five and eight years after the birth of their first child, they tended to be undereducated, underemployed and continued to have further children. Six months after the birth of their first child, most of the mothers were lacking in knowledge about parenting and displayed problematic parenting styles. By the time the children were 8 years old, 38% of the mothers were depressed. Many of the sample were at risk of abusing or neglecting their children, in part as a result of their lack of readiness for the parenting role. They were found to be more intolerant, insensitive and punitive, and less verbal than adult mothers. Although their infants were healthy at birth, assessments at 1, 3, 5, 8 and 10 years of age revealed problems, including insecure attachment, language delays, internalizing and externalizing behaviours and underachievement at school.

Box 8.2 indicates some of the main health risks that are faced by young women who become pregnant during adolescence.

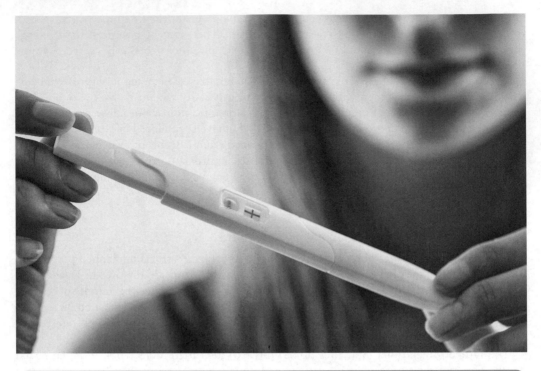

Peter Cade/Getty images

Social and health risks involved in teenage pregnancy (adapted from Frances, 2010)

Babies born to teenage mothers have worse health outcomes than those of older mothers since they are:

- More likely to be born prematurely or at a low birth weight;
- 60% more likely to die in the first year of life than babies of mothers aged 20–39;
- Twice as likely to be admitted to hospital as a result of an accident or gastroenteritis.

Teenage mothers have specific problems. They are:

- Three times more likely to get post-natal depression than older mothers;
- At a higher risk of poor mental health for three years after the birth;

- Three times more likely to smoke during pregnancy than mothers over 35 years;
- One-third less likely to breastfeed;
- Likely to struggle to complete education and find it difficult to gain employment.

However, as Borkowski *et al.* (2007) discovered, a proportion of the young mothers *were* resilient and experienced positive growth during their transition to adulthood, for example, through educational attainment, employment, self-esteem and effective parenting practices. The researchers found several main factors that identified resilience in this group. It was important for the mothers to have family support from their own parents. Grandmothers in particular played an important role in providing nurturance, financial support and stability for the child. Usually the child's father was not resident with the mother, but where the father maintained some form of contact with the child, that factor resulted in improved emotional well-being in the children. His continued positive involvement during adolescence was a protective factor against psychological distress in the child. The social environment could also provide protection. Social competence increased when the children were involved in some form of community activity. Religious affiliation appeared to promote resilience by providing positive role models and helping the children's identity development through commitment to belief systems and the encouragement of prosocial behaviour. The researchers concluded that, even in deprived neighbourhoods, there were a range of protective mechanisms that could promote the resilience both of the teenage mothers and of their children.

Interventions to reduce and prevent teenage pregnancy

Over the past decade there has been some progress in reducing the number of teenage pregnancies in that England's under-18 pregnancy rate is at its lowest level for 20 years (Frances, 2010). The rate of under-18 conceptions fell by 13% between 1998 and 2008. Additionally, the birth rate arising from under-18 conceptions fell by 25% during that period. The discrepancy between conceptions and actual births can be explained by the increase in terminations, indicating that early childbearing has become less appealing to young women. The reduction in under-18 conceptions can also be attributed to the success of interventions to prevent teenage pregnancy and risky sexual behaviour. School- and college-based contraceptive and sexual health services (CASH) have increased. In schools, trained teachers, support staff and nurses deliver PSHE and initiatives such as Sex and Relationship Education (SRE). These programmes aim to give children and young people knowledge and social skills to resist pressures from the peer group, partners and the media to engage in unwanted sexual activity and to understand issues like sexual consent, responsibility and safer sex. Working in single-gender groups to discuss SRE is found to be a useful initial way of meeting the needs of both young women and young men. However, it is also essential that young people of both genders encounter each other to learn about their different needs and perspectives and to engage in discussion.

> Box 8.3

Evaluation of the Teens and Toddlers Project (adapted from Cater & McDowell, 2010)

Teens and Toddlers is a teenage pregnancy prevention programme which aims to heighten awareness in young people aged 14–16 years of the reality of conception and parenthood long before pregnancy occurs. The programme gives opportunities for at-risk young people to interact with 3–5-year-olds during a twice-weekly two-hour session in a safe nursery environment followed by an hour of discussion and reflection on the experience. The three elements of the programme include: one-to-one contact between the adolescent and a toddler; tuition on child development, parenting skills, sex education and relationships; counselling for those young people considered to be most at risk. The benefits to participants are:

- Prevention of teenage pregnancy;
- Learning good communication skills;
- Developing emotional literacy, self-reflection and self-management skills;
- Learning about parenting and caring for toddlers;
- Engaging with the wider community;
- Discovering possible career opportunities in childcare;
- Creating a sense of achievement;
- Developing alternative life-goals to early parenthood, such as education and career opportunities.

Interviews with participants reveal the impact of the programme on attitudes towards parenthood. Here James, one of the participating boys, evaluates the programme:

> It's good for making boys think about babies and how you want to be there for them and not just be a father but be a proper dad instead. And you can't always be there for them when you're like a teenager, so it's bound to work out better if you leave it 'til you're older and you've got a job and stuff . . . I think I learnt that you just don't think like, when you're in the moment [laughs] that it could just be that one time. And you shouldn't always take the girl's word for it that she's on the pill, cos some girls trick you. Just like girls shouldn't always trust boys. And then what are you gonna do? So if you're gonna use them you should, like, use them all the time.
>
> (ibid.)

Currently, there is support for teenage parents through social programmes such as Care to Learn, a scheme for helping young parents continue with their education, and initiatives such as Family Nurse Partnership which provide young mothers and their partners with parenting classes. Education that focuses on the importance of relationships rather than simply on the biological facts is more likely to enable young people to achieve positive attitudes towards sexual health and to be more confident in being responsible about behaviour within sexual and romantic relationships. Education can also help young women to develop effective communication skills, including the capacity to deal with unwanted peer pressure to engage in sexual behaviour. Most importantly, education programmes can provide knowledge about methods for protecting against unintended pregnancy, sexually transmitted infections and HIV/AIDS.

Preventing teenage pregnancy is about increasing awareness and knowledge as well as building up self-esteem, aspirations and confidence. Professionals need to be confident in talking about sexual matters with young people, for example, about contraception, including emergency contraception, and in equipping young people with the negotiating skills to resist peer pressure to engage in sexual activity before they are ready. It is important to involve young men too and to be ready to discuss such topics as dating violence. There is unequal provision of SRE and in some communities parents object on the grounds that their children are not yet sexually active (Vydelingum & Colliety, 2011), leading to difficult ethical dilemmas for educators and sexual health advisors.

CASE STUDY 8.4

How appropriate is sex education for children?

Bushra is 13 years old. Her parents were horrified when they discovered that the school had invited a sexual health adviser to deliver a series of lessons on choice with regard to sexual relationships. Since they believed strongly that young people should not engage in sexual behaviour before marriage, they planned to withdraw her on principle from all such lessons. Bushra herself wanted to attend the lessons and hated the idea of being different from the rest of her peer group.

Discussion questions

Should the school respect the parents' wishes on this matter? Should Bushra be consulted on whether she wishes to learn about safer sex?

There is a tension between providing appropriate sex and relationship education for young people and showing respect for culturally sensitive issues. As Vydelingum and Colliety (2011) point out, some Christian, Hindu and Muslim parents may find it unacceptable that their teenage children should be receiving sex education at school since, in their view, the young people are not yet sexually active and so are in no need of being protected against sexually transmitted infections or unplanned pregnancy.

Chapter summary

Young people are becoming sexually active at an earlier age. The chapter explores typical sexual development and considers risk factors associated with harmful sexual behaviour. It also examines outcomes resulting from unprotected sex, such as unplanned pregnancy and sexually transmitted infections. The UK has one of the highest rates of teenage pregnancy in Europe but there is evidence that the rates are decreasing. The chapter looks at some interventions to heighten young people's awareness of risks and to change attitudes in such areas as partner violence.

Discussion points

- There is an increase in partner violence among young people. What can be done to alter this disturbing trend?
- Why does the UK have one of the highest rates of teenage pregnancy in Europe?
- How can educators reach an ethical decision about the age at which young people should be offered appropriate sexual health advice and information?

Further reading

See: Borkowski, J. (ed.) (2007) *Risk and Resilience: Adolescent Mothers and Their Children Grow Up*, London: Routledge, for a sensitive account of the relationship between young mothers and their children.

Websites and resources

An excellent free resource with accompanying DVD which addresses sexual bullying and gender conflict among young people is: Jennifer, D. & Williams, S. (2011) *Linking Lies*, London: Lewisham College. Can be downloaded from:
   www.lsis.org.uk

Brook offer guidance on sexual health and on teenage pregnancy:
   http://www.brook.org.uk/

Websites designed to be user-friendly for young people include:
www.afraidtoask.com and www.sexworthtalkingabout.co.uk

A website created by Patrick Carnes containing useful advice and resources to help individuals affected by sexual addiction and compulsive sexual behaviour is:
www.sexhelp.com

The Teenage Pregnancy Independent Advisory Group provides useful information for nurses, health visitors and midwives on teenage pregnancy and strategies for addressing the issue and supporting young parents:
http://webarchive.nationalarchives.gov.uk/20100418065544/dcsf.gov.uk/everychildmatters/healthandwellbeing/teenagepregnancy/tpiag/tpiag/

The Brandon Centre for Counselling and Psychotherapy for Young People is a charitable organization that has existed for over 40 years. Originally called the London Youth Advisory Centre (LYAC), it was started as a contraceptive service for young women aged 12 to 25 years.

The founder, Dr Faith Spicer, recognized that young women needed to have access to a service that allowed them time to talk through emotional issues that accompanied requests for contraception. Shortly after the founding of the contraceptive service an information service and a psychotherapy service were initiated for young women and young men due to the scale of the emotional needs of young people in the local community and beyond. These services were made accessible by allowing self-referral and confidentiality, by providing comfortable, welcoming and 'non-institutional premises' in the heart of the local community and by receptionists being friendly without being intrusive.
http://www.brandon-centre.org.uk/

Chapter 9

Emotional health and well-being

> **Map of the chapter**
>
> This chapter examines the risk and protective processes involved in child and adolescent emotional health and well-being. It considers the perspectives of young people on common mental health difficulties and the stigma that surrounds them. It looks at the role of peer support in helping to overcome prejudice and ignorance about mental health issues. Then it describes the internalization of emotional and behavioural difficulties, in depression and anxiety, and their externalization through aggressive and disruptive behaviour. The chapter ends by discussing a school-based intervention to support the transition of vulnerable young people from primary to secondary school.

As indicated in earlier chapters, parents/carers play a crucial role in the emotional health and well-being of children and young people. As indicated in Chapter 3, if children's needs are not met, then social, emotional and cognitive processes are put at risk. Case Study 9.1 gives an example of the success of early intervention in preventing later emotional and behavioural difficulties in a child whose refugee mother, Magda, was under so much stress that she was not relating well to her child, Yuri. Magda had experienced large-scale disruption in her own life and this had affected her capacity to use appropriate parenting skills. Through the therapeutic use of video, Magda was enabled to reconnect with her emotions of loving and caring.

Using video feedback as an early intervention (adapted from Balbernie & Gorney, 2011)

Video feedback can be a very effective way of intervening early in order to facilitate change in the ways in which parents relate to their children. The Keys to Interactive Parenting Scale (KIPS) rates video material gained from observing parents and their children interact with one another. This approach provides a useful combination of assessment and service-monitoring and provides a profile of the strengths and areas of potential growth which can then be immensely helpful in guiding parents to think constructively about their parenting skills. The observable behaviour and the dynamics of the parent-child relationship are present on video and can then be discussed and reflected on in a supportive setting. Balbernie and Gorney (ibid.) give a vivid example. Magda, from Belarus, wanted help because she reported that she lacked positive feelings towards her son, Yuri. She found him very difficult to manage and the very sight of him caused her to feel stressed. She had in the past smacked him so severely that he was bruised and feared that she might do this again. She told the therapist that she had experienced a very difficult childhood herself. The therapist edited the video clips that he had made of Magda playing with Yuri so that she could watch herself parenting. Observation of the video would form the basis of the therapeutic work. Magda was able to watch a scene of herself playing Lego with Yuri in which she created a safe space for him to explore his game and so to increase his confidence. The therapist commented on her skill at playing alongside Yuri and encouraged Magda to admit that she was doing something good with her child. When the therapist invited Magda to name what she was doing, she eventually said, 'being patient'. The therapist asked her if anyone had been patient like that with her as a child and she recalled that her grandmother was. The therapist and Magda discussed these memories of the grandmother and then continued to explore times when she could be patient with Yuri. The edited video material provided a clear focus on actual behaviour that had positive outcomes. The dynamics of the parent-child relationship could then be discussed and then built upon for future parenting. In addition, the KIPS method provides a way of evaluating the effectiveness of the intervention over a period of time. Typically, parents' scores start low and then rise as they participate in therapeutic interventions. The sessions always culminate with the therapist giving the parents the final DVD as a souvenir of them and their child together. Often the DVD is shown to other family members who then provide commentary and positive feedback.

Discussion questions

Why was this intervention successful? Would the effects last?

Case Study 9.1 illustrates the value of parenting support early in the child's life to prevent later abuse and neglect. With children older than Yuri, it becomes increasingly important to consult with them about the issues that are causing them distress and to involve them in identifying solutions. Most children have great reserves of resilience but need to be given opportunities to take responsibility in age-appropriate ways, and given relevant information that will enable them to make informed choices about their own lives. Just as Magda responded to the opportunity to reflect on her own relationships and her own family history, so children and young people need to be given opportunities and support to deal with the inevitable conflicts and disruptions in relationships that they will meet in their lives.

Perspectives of children and young people

Children and young people with emotional and behavioural difficulties frequently report that they feel excluded and ignored at school, and that their social and emotional needs are not met. Consequently, they often become disengaged from school through misbehaviour, withdrawal or absenteeism. They are often labelled as failures and are at risk of being bullied by peers (Toynbee, 2009). The sense of shame and embarrassment that surrounds the concept of mental health difficulty can contribute to the fact that young people's social, emotional and behavioural issues are often unrecognized or even denied.

YoungMinds (2010) conducted a stigma survey among 2,700 young people aged 9–16 years. The participants revealed that more than 50% of them had heard vulnerable peers being called abusive names, such as 'weirdo', 'retard', 'idiot', 'freak', 'schizo', 'crazy' or 'psycho'. Twenty-five per cent reported that it was easier to tell someone about being physically ill than about feeling mentally distressed. As part of the Royal College of Psychiatrists Anti-Stigma campaign, Gale and Holling (2000) ran a series of focus groups among young people from disadvantaged backgrounds to find out what these young people needed to know about mental health and how they would like it to be presented. There were three key findings:

- The young people's knowledge and understanding of mental health issues was very low;
- They lacked an appropriate emotional language to express themselves adequately about mental health difficulties;
- Their limited knowledge and understanding, and their lack of emotional language, was in spite of their proximity with the experience of mental illness in family members or friends.

For example, in combination, the words 'mental', 'health' and 'problem' did not promote much discussion in the focus groups. By contrast, words like 'nutter', 'weirdo' and 'psycho' were meaningful and suggested a wide range of behaviours and feelings. Young people in the focus groups stated that such words implied being 'out of control' or 'unusual' or 'having a disability'. However, Box 9.1 indicates the value of using young people's vocabulary for describing emotional distress and listening to their accounts of the coping strategies that they adopt.

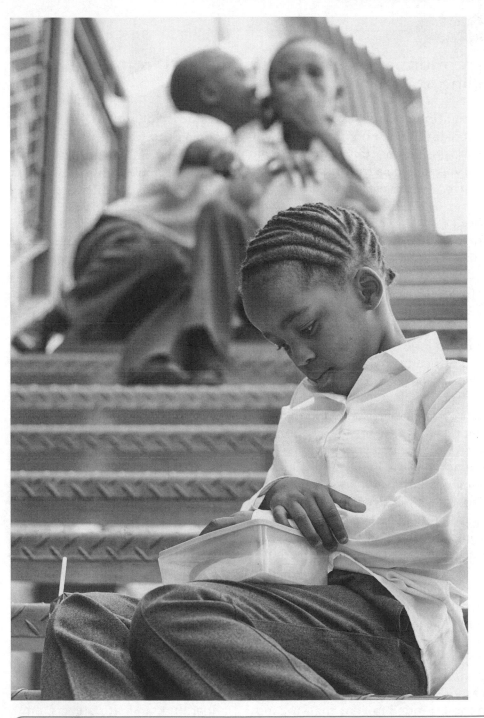

2A Images/Getty images

Box 9.1

Perceptions of mental health (adapted from Gale & Holling, 2000)

Gale and Holling (ibid.) carried out a 16-month study exploring the attitudes and perceptions of a broad range of young people aged from 12 to 14 years towards positive mental health and mental illness. The main sample consisted of 170 young people from a variety of social and ethnic minority backgrounds who attended mainstream schools in rural, suburban and inner-city areas of Scotland. The researchers used focus group discussions and individual interviews to elicit the young people's attitudes. The main categories elicited from these discussions were presented under five headings: understanding of positive mental health; what might make young people feel mentally healthy and unhealthy; how other people might promote young people's mental health; their own strategies for dealing with their own negative feelings; perceived differences between themselves and adults:

- *Positive mental health*: Young people from less advantaged backgrounds had difficulty in defining the term 'mentally healthy'; those from suburban schools and those from minority ethnic backgrounds referred to it as 'the absence of illness' or in terms of happiness and confidence. For some, the term was equated with 'normality' but the young people found it hard to define what they meant by normality.
- *What might make young people feel mentally healthy and unhealthy*: Key elements were: family and friends; having someone to talk to; personal achievement; feeling good about yourself.
- *Promoting positive mental health*: A key theme was the role of adults to help young people feel safe, both physically and emotionally. These adults could be parents but other adults could also fill this role. Many of the participants felt that there were no professionals that they could really trust, though they specifically mentioned ChildLine as a valuable service that could be used for confidential matters. Those from ethnic minority backgrounds felt strongly that personal issues should not be discussed outside the family and that, on issues which could not be discussed with parents, members of the extended family (often close to them in age) were appropriate people to approach.
- *Dealing with negative feelings*: There were two main categories of response: reactions to angry feelings and reactions to sadness. Young people tended to vent their feelings of anger on inanimate objects, on siblings or on peers, through aggressive acts, such as fighting; there were few behavioural differences between boys and girls but the boys discussed their aggression openly in the focus groups while the girls disclosed them

privately on self-completion forms. Feelings of sadness, by contrast, were dealt with through internalization. Suicidal thoughts were discussed by one group; some described eating or sleeping; others spoke of talking to a trusted other, including a professional, as a coping strategy. Counselling was perceived positively by some as active coping but by others as a stigma.

- *Perceived differences between themselves and adults:* All the participants identified precipitating factors common to both adults and young people, for example, the death of friends and relatives, falling out with people and stress. However, factors distinctive for adults included: job insecurity, financial concerns and worries about children. By contrast, young people's issues were often described as less important than those of adults.

Discussion questions

How could these young people be helped to evaluate the effectiveness or otherwise of their coping strategies? How could teachers and healthcare professionals build on the resilience shown by the young people themselves?

The young people in this study demonstrated a range of coping strategies, some effective (such as sharing a difficulty), others avoidant (such as denying the problem, sleeping or drinking alcohol). The authors concluded that the term 'mental health' did not appear to have much meaning for young people in this study and recommended the use of a different vocabulary in educational or therapeutic work with young people.

The findings confirm the Mental Health Foundation's inquiry into the emotional well-being of children and young people who were users of mental health services (MHF, 1999). Some respondents said that it was hard for them to access services and that they found the professionals intimidating or apparently uncaring. Some also found it embarrassing or awkward to be asked too quickly to disclose details about distressing incidents in their lives. However, many *were* satisfied with the quality of the care that they received. They appreciated being listened to and cared for, especially when the professionals were flexible and informal. The report also recommended that schools could play a significant part in promoting children's mental health through the recognition and implementation of social and emotional education in all aspects of the curriculum and in the life of the school (see the discussion of the SEAL curriculum in Chapter 2). Counteracting the effects of stigma would be a key aspect of such activity.

In the context of overcoming stigma, there is great potential in the use of peer support methods. Box 9.2 indicates the potential of peer support in complementing the work of professionals to help young people readjust to the peer group following a time of emotional vulnerability. Such young people benefit from the support of adults, for example, the pastoral care teams at school, but they can also benefit from encounters with other young people who have shared similar difficulties. The example in Box 9.2 is **obsessive compulsive disorder (OCD)** but the issues raised could be applied to other areas where children and young people experience emotional and behavioural difficulties. An OCD is a common mental health problem with symptoms that include recurring obsessive thoughts and accompanying repetitive compulsions, such as thinking obsessively about germs and dirt and so feeling compelled to wash hands repeatedly in order to become clean.

Box 9.2

The role of peer support (adapted from Kröger, 2010)

Kröger (ibid.) examined the impact that having an OCD can have on young people's social interactions with peers. She interviewed five young people, aged from 14 to 18 years, who no longer required psychological therapy for their illness. She identified four main themes:

- *The stigma of having OCD*: The young people reported fear of rejection by others and deep feelings of shame and embarrassment about their condition. The participants in this research said that they were afraid of being perceived as 'weird', 'crazy' or 'a freak'.
- *The impact on social life*: They also reported that they often distanced themselves from others because of their preoccupation with their compulsions. As a result, they were likely to become lonely and isolated from their peers.
- *Being controlled by the disorder*: They experienced a great deal of misery and powerlessness as they felt that the OCD controlled their lives. None of them had actually known another person with the same disorder and wished that they could have shared their experiences with a peer.
- *Peer support*: They indicated that, now that they had recovered, they would appreciate the chance to offer peer support to others in the same situation. This could help the other person and also increase their own confidence and incentive to stay well. They believed that the sharing of personal experience could play a strong role in aiding recovery.

Discussion questions

What are some of the barriers that prevent recovered young people from offering peer support? How useful might this kind of peer support be in reducing prejudice towards young people with a mental health difficulty?

Kröger (2010) concludes that there is a need for clinicians to develop a better understanding of the difficulties that young people face around the stigma of having a mental health difficulty. Meeting a recovered young person could, she argues, provide an inspirational role model for others and increase the motivation to persist with treatment, despite the difficulties.

There are many examples of young people in distress being supported by their peers. Peer tutoring is one method that has very positive outcomes. For example, Classwide Peer Tutoring (CWPT) involves all students in a class, including those with social and emotional difficulties, in the learning process. It is a good example of cooperative learning since students rely on one another's achievements in order to improve their own. There is also the opportunity to engage actively in learning through questioning, instructing, reinforcing and praising accurate responses to questions. Karagiannakis and Sladeczek (2009) report on a study evaluating the impact of CWPT on the attainment and self-concept of children with emotional and behavioural difficulties. The class was divided into two teams that engaged in competitions for 1–2 weeks. Following a highly structured teacher-developed lesson, the pupils tutored one another on the same materials. The peer tutors were trained to reinforce correct responses and to correct errors in a supportive way. Each pair accumulated points for their team. At the end of the 1- or 2-week competition, the students were given a test to assess what they had learned. Each team's points were added and the winning team announced. The researchers observed significant improvements in the on-task behaviour of students with emotional and behavioural difficulties who participated in CWPT. All who participated reported that they enjoyed the experience, not least the fact that the approach was completely inclusive.

Internalizing and externalizing behaviour

Emotional and behavioural difficulties are commonly divided into two major categories: those that *internalize* the difficulty and those that *externalize* it. A young person who internalizes these difficulties tends to become anxious, fearful or depressed, or develops physical complaints or an eating disorder or avoids school. The **internalizing of mental health difficulties** is related long term to low self-esteem, anxiety and depression. Young people who **externalize emotional difficulties** act them out, for example, in conduct disorders and attention deficit and hyper-activity disorder (ADHD). Drug and alcohol abuse can be both a cause and an outcome of emotional and behavioural difficulty. Those with externalizing disorders are often seen as disaffected or disruptive.The stresses that many young people experience in areas of high poverty and deprivation can increase the risk.

A minority of young people with mental health problems will be referred to and receive help from Child and Adolescent Mental Health Services (CAMHS). Rutter *et al.* (2006) found that only 10–21% of children with mental health problems received professional help. The majority were left to deal with their difficulties on their own or with support from those around them: their family; friends; teachers; social workers. Counselling and psychotherapy demonstrate the value of concentrating on the quality of relationships. Therapy offers a safe space in which the child or young person can begin to reflect on the aspects of life that worry them. Counselling can provide a constructive way for children and young people to view their problems in new ways and to find practical ways of changing their behaviour, as is indicated in Case Study 9.2.

CASE STUDY 9.2

Mack: a boy with emotional needs

Mack, aged 8, was identified by his teachers as a child with emotional and behavioural difficulties which, in their view, stemmed from his unhappy home life. Since his father left home, Mack had found it hard to concentrate and was frequently involved in disputes with his classmates. Because of his tantrums and unpredictable outbursts, he had very few friends and often spent time on his own. He was referred to CAMHS, where the therapist spent time addressing his relationship difficulties within the family. Mack was very reluctant to talk about his thoughts and feelings so the therapist used small model figures as props for him to enact some of the difficulties that Mack was experiencing at home. Using these figures to represent different members of his family, Mack was able to express his anxiety and his feelings of rejection by his Dad. He also enacted some of the arguments that had happened between his parents as they separated over a period of some months. His mother, Tracey, said that she had found it very difficult to talk to Mack because of his 'moodiness'. The therapist explained that she could offer them a solution-focused approach to their difficulties; there were particular areas that they could work on together. She asked where each would like to begin. Mack said that he wished his mother could spend more time with him. Tracey said that she wanted to have more fun with Mack as they used to do. In the safety of the counselling room, they each practised new ways of behaving towards each other. Tracey practised thanking Mack when he did something positive instead of shouting at him when he was moody. Mack was able to say directly that he had hated the arguments and missed his Dad. The therapist set goals for them at the end of each session. Over time, Tracey reported that there were fewer arguments at home as she became less tense. Mack became calmer at school and he started to form friendships with other boys in his class.

Discussion questions

Was play therapy the best way to enable Mack to express his feelings? Are there alternative ways in which the therapist might have worked on the family relationships? Should Mack's Dad have been involved too?

The following sections describe a range of emotional and behavioural difficulties commonly experienced by children and young people. The next sections also include examples from a range of helpful interventions.

Depression and anxiety

Depression is one of the commonest mental health disorders among children and young people, and is indicated by such aspects as persistent feelings of sadness, inability to concentrate, apathy, withdrawal from social interaction, lack of interest in people and activities, low self-esteem, suicidal thoughts. Eating patterns can also be affected. Rutter (2000) identified the following risk factors for depression:

- *Family factors:* violence, abuse, neglect in the family; abusive, violent relationships; being a young person looked after outside the family; a history of mental illness in the family; death and loss in the family; rejection by parents.
- *Social factors:* poverty; deprivation; homelessness; rejection by peers; social exclusion; being a member of a deviant peer group.
- *Factors within the individual child or young person:* chronic physical illness; communication difficulties; deafness; academic failure; under-age sexual activity.

Suicidal thoughts and feelings of hopelessness are characteristic of depression. Self-harming behaviour, for example, cutting oneself, is more common among girls than boys and also occurs more frequently among young people with low self-esteem and inadequate coping strategies (Cowie *et al.*, 2004). Suicide is a leading cause of death among young people, with boys and young men being especially at risk. Eskin (1995) investigated young people's attitudes towards suicide and a suicidal classmate among 98 girl and 69 boy Swedish high-school students. Among the Swedish students, more boys than girls said that people have the right to commit suicide and that suicide can be a solution to some problems. More girls than boys expressed a belief in life after death.

Anxiety disorders include *general anxiety* (for example, general feelings of unease and uncertainty about self-image or body image, or anxiety about examination performance), **separation anxiety** (expressed by excessive clinging to parents or school refusal), *phobias* (associated with somatic symptoms, such as sweating, diarrhoea and panic attacks) including *obsessive compulsive disorders* (OCDs), social phobia and panic disorders. Around 3–8% of the child population experiences phobias which are more extreme and persistent forms of anxiety. A characteristic of phobias is that they often lead to a compulsive avoidance of the feared situation or object. Many childhood phobias are simply outgrown by the time of adolescence but can be very distressing to the young person and their family while they exist. There can be specific triggers for anxiety. In the case of *school phobia* – or refusal to go to school – it may be that the child or young person is being bullied, or that they are extremely stressed and anxious about some aspect of their academic performance (Chamberlain *et al.*, 2011). Often there is an accumulation of different factors which become overwhelming.

There are a number of ways of working with fears and phobias, including:

- *Desensitization:* Here the child is taught to relax and is then gradually exposed to the situation or object that they fear. Once relaxed, the child, with the help of the therapist, imagines themselves in the anxiety-provoking situation. When they are ready to imagine themselves in that situation without feeling anxious, the therapist moves on to increased exposure to the source of the phobia.
- *Emotive imagery:* This approach uses narrative to develop images which produce anxiety-reducing emotions, like pride, competence and assertiveness. Positive images are used within a narrative that involves episodes in the child's life. Gradually the anxiety-producing images are introduced into the narrative. The positive images enable the child to control feelings of fear.

- *Cognitive approaches:* These approaches build on the interactions among feelings, thoughts and behaviour. Most anxieties are irrational so this approach challenges the irrational aspects of the child's cognitions. The child then learns logical self-statements which replace the irrational ones and support more reasonable beliefs.

As discussed in Chapter 3, there is continuity in the characteristics of attachment behaviour, especially when there is a perceived threat to the attachment bond. Case Study 9.3 illustrates how a seemingly secure child could become extremely anxious and revert to attachment behaviours more typical of a toddler. Her separation anxiety was expressed through excessive clinging to her mother.

CASE STUDY 9.3

Maisie: a child with separation anxiety

Maisie was an apparently happy, outgoing 9-year-old who loved school and had many friends. Suddenly, she showed great reluctance to go to school and would no longer walk with her friends in the mornings. Her mother accompanied her in the mornings in order to reassure her but Maisie clung to her and began having panic attacks the nearer they got to the school gate. At home, she became very anxious at night and refused to sleep unless the hall light was left on. She no longer wanted to stay overnight with relatives or friends. She needed to stay close to her mother. The GP referred Maisie and her mother to a psychologist who adopted a **Cognitive Behavioural Therapy (CBT)** approach to treatment. In this case, Kate, the therapist, explained to Maisie and her mother how anxiety affects the body, the mind and emotions. She encouraged Maisie's mother to be open about Maisie's fears and to feel free to talk about them with her. She encouraged Maisie's mother to think about how Maisie's thoughts were influencing the way she responded to situations when she had to be separated from her mother. Together, the psychologist, Maisie and her mother identified achievable goals, for example, walking to school without feeling anxious, and specific tasks, such as Maisie letting go of her mother's hand as they neared the school gate. Over time, Maisie became able to walk to school with one close friend. Later, she resumed occasional overnight stays with close friends and relatives. The therapeutic intervention helped her to overcome her anxiety and she became the happy child that she had been before.

Discussion question

The therapist focused on Maisie's symptoms and behaviour. Might other approaches that explored the underlying reasons for Maisie's separation anxiety have been more appropriate?

Cognitive approaches have a high success rate in the treatment of anxiety disorders as described in Case Study 9.3. Some clinicians, however, argue that cognitive approaches are best used in conjunction with methods that explore the underlying causes of the anxiety.

Aggressive and disruptive behaviours

Thousands of pupils are excluded from school each year for a variety of reasons, mostly related to aggressive and disruptive behaviour. There are many factors that underlie disturbances in children's behaviour. These include:

- Death of a parent or close family member;
- Parental separation or divorce;
- Illness or injury;
- Adjusting to new family members (reconstituted family);
- Birth of a sibling;
- Parental discord or domestic violence;
- Family member leaves home;
- Change of schools;
- A close friend moves away;
- Stress from tests and examinations;
- Being bullied at school.

Additionally, risks come from certain environments. In some inner-city estates, there is a heightened risk of experiencing violent, aggressive behaviour (e.g., in lifts, on public transport, in walkways, on the street) in the course of going about everyday activities.

Arnold *et al.* (2009), in a phenomenological analysis of children and young people excluded from school for disruptive behaviour, identified the strong impact of adverse family circumstances, such as marital breakdown or domestic violence. In each case, the family was undergoing a period of significant instability, and the child's emotional and behavioural difficulties usually coincided with its onset. Family instability and environmental disadvantage alone did not explain the young person's difficulties but certainly provided added risk factors. There are always reasons for the disruptive behaviour, often linked to some current or past experience. For example, the process of relinquishing parents as attachment figures usually begins in early adolescence when young people develop the concept of their parents as people they love, but also come to understand that parents cannot always guarantee security. Case Study 9.4 describes the attachment issues precipitated by family discord just as Maggie was about to make the transition from primary to secondary school. The combination of circumstances and the ways in which they were handled resulted in Maggie being labelled as a disruptive pupil.

Maggie: a disruptive pupil

Maggie had no major difficulties while she was at primary school. She was a sociable girl who enjoyed class work, sports and music. She made lots of friends from school and through her involvement in teams and in the school brass band. When Maggie was 11, during the transition to secondary school, her parents started to have serious arguments, some of which escalated into violence. At the same time she reached puberty and suddenly looked very mature for her age. Her mother found her increasingly difficult to manage at home. Maggie refused to help out in any way and often had noisy tantrums when challenged. She refused to eat meals and preferred to snack on junk foods in her bedroom. She would often leave the house angrily and not return for hours. Her mother suspected that she was drinking alcohol in the park with young people who congregated there. Maggie always denied this.

By the time Maggie was 12, her parents had separated and subsequently divorced. There was a protracted legal battle over custody and access. Maggie felt torn between Mum and Dad and longed for them all to be back together again as a family. But she hated visiting her Dad and his new partner and, after a few weeks, refused to go to his house. Her very best friend went to a different secondary school so Maggie felt that she had no one in whom she could confide. She found the teachers much stricter than those in her primary school. She often dreamed about being back in Year 6. From the beginning, her behaviour in Year 7 was difficult. She rebelled against the rules and frequently clashed with her teachers. Her behaviour in class deteriorated so that she was regularly sent out for being disruptive. Lunchtime supervisors also complained about her behaviour in the lunch queue. This led to a series of detentions which she resented very much. She had two fixed-term suspensions and the school warned her parents that a permanent exclusion was likely.

Discussion questions

Was exclusion the most appropriate way of dealing with Maggie? What alternative interventions might have worked? How important was home-school liaison in Maggie's case?

Working with vulnerable young people

Developing appropriate emotional support for children and adolescents is a challenging task. Difficulties include the actual location of services, the approach adopted by professionals working in multidisciplinary teams, and attitudes of young people and their families towards mental health issues. It is often the 'little things' that make a difference – the care and attention shown by staff in everyday interactions with the young people in their care (Smith & Cowie, 2010). Positive staff attitudes are very important. In everyday life, professionals and parents need to be alert to the potential presence of negative attitudes towards vulnerable children and young people with special needs. Training should include knowledge about child development and about the outcomes that stigma can have, if not challenged, on children's self-esteem (Naylor *et al.*, 2009).

It is essential to create a caring climate in schools and to have adults who are prepared to be significant others to the children and young people in their care. Box 9.3 gives an example of how one school, Acland Burghley School, involved staff and peer supporters in a Head Start programme, designed to ease the transition of vulnerable students from primary to secondary school. Acland Burghley is a mixed, inner-city comprehensive school with over 1,200 students, including a sixth form. Twenty-two per cent of students are identified as having special educational needs and disability (SEND) and 24% have English as a second language (EAL). The school had 34% of students who were eligible for free school meals (FSM) and there was an upward trend in numbers, with 46% FSM for the Year 7 intake for September 2011. The school has significantly more boys than girls, with a 2:1 ratio of boys to girls. The school wanted to ensure that vulnerable Year 6 students were supported so that they could cope with the transition from primary to secondary school. The target students for this support were students on the autistic spectrum, students with speech and language difficulties, children with learning difficulties, students on the child protection register and students with poor attendance. The Head Start project had the following aims:

- Alleviating anxiety and developing confidence to cope with secondary transition;
- Preparing SEND students for the new routines of secondary school and familiarizing them with the workings of the Year 7 timetable;
- Supporting students in finding their way around the school;
- Providing an opportunity for students to meet relevant members of staff;
- Giving students the opportunity to experience secondary lessons;
- Organizing for students to meet and work with 'ABC Peer Supporters' who would continue to support them in Year 7;
- Helping students develop new relationships with their peers.

Because of the success of this programme, other schools in the locality have asked for guidance in developing a similar scheme and the Acland Burghley team, including the peer supporters, have been happy to share their expertise.

Box 9.3

The Acland Burghley Head Start programme: supporting vulnerable Year 6 students with their primary to secondary school transition (adapted with permission from Vavi Hillel, Head Start Programme Leader, Acland Burghley School)

The Head Start programme is designed to provide additional support for vulnerable Year 6 students in addition to the school's planned induction day for all incoming Year 7 students held at the end of June every year. The Head Start programme normally takes place two weeks before the Year 7 induction day in June. Once the school knows which students will be attending Acland Burghley in Year 7, letters are sent to all their schools asking the schools to identify all the students on their school's special needs register who might be vulnerable at the time of transition to secondary school and who might benefit from extra support in addition to the induction day. Schools are sent referral forms and are asked to identify the area of concern or difficulty and to provide any relevant medical information. Once Acland Burghley receives the referrals from primary schools, as Head Start Programme Leader I select students in consultation with the primary schools. The parents and carers of selected students are written to and informed that their child's primary school has recommended their child for the programme. They receive an information leaflet which outlines the aims and content of the programme and they are asked to sign a consent form. In June 2011, the school selected 13 students to take part in the programme. I deliver the programme with the help of a learning support assistant, the head of Year 7, an art teacher and a team of ABC Peer Supporters. In preparation for the Head Start programme, ABC Peer Supporters are matched to Head Start students and if possible to those who attended their same primary school. They receive a two-hour training session which provides them with an overview of the Head Start programme, information about the programme activities, training on listening skills and leading group activities and a chance to practise their roles. Peer Supporters also get a chance to find out about the Year 6 student who they will be supporting. Peer supporters receive training on autistic spectrum disorders (ASD) from the head of the ASD unit in the school. In some instances, Peer Supporters have actually participated in the Head Start programme when they were in Year 6.

The identified Year 6 students are invited to spend two mornings at Acland Burghley in mid-June and they take part in a programme of planned activities, while also having the chance to attend Acland Burghley when the rest of the school community is present. Students work with their Year 6 peers and Peer

Supporters and engage in fun and informative activities which are designed to help them understand the school layout, routines and expectations as well as helping them make friendships with their peers and Peer Supporter.

At the end of the two days all the Year 6 students are given a gift of a pencil case with all the equipment they will need for secondary school and a folder containing the work they have produced during the two mornings. They also receive a certificate and a photograph of the whole group including the Peer Supporters and staff. Parents and carers are invited to attend an evening meeting during the two-day programme. This meeting gives the parents and carers an opportunity to get to know other parents and the opportunity to talk about their child and any issues they want to raise. Parents' concerns are recorded and followed up by the school. Here is a representative comment from one of the Peer Supporters:

Year 9 Peer Supporter

'From the moment they arrived you could sense the enthusiasm growing inside them, as they began making friends with one another and they had infinite questions to ask about the school. Their excitement only increased throughout the day as they began to feel more like a community and included in the school.'

Many activities are arranged for the new students, some to be done as individuals and others in groups to increase their socializing skills. These activities include: creative writing; passing around your favourite object and giving a description; an activity worksheet about the student/Peer Supporter; and the favourite of most students, the Year 6s are given a map and told to find certain rooms in the school. This activity is based on the idea of exploring and finding your own way around the school building. On the Head Start days students are introduced to the head teacher, SENCO and the Head of Year 7. Overall it was a great day for everyone.

One Year 6 student said, 'We enjoyed showing our favourite toy', and another commented that 'The Peer Supporters did a very good job. I'm so excited about coming to Acland Burghley; I'm even looking forward to getting lost!'

It was wonderful to see how their confidence grew throughout the two sessions as they were running around, already part of the Acland Burghley community.

Head Start students and Peer Supporters complete a questionnaire giving feedback on the two-day programme and Head Start students give feedback on the difference that it has made for their transition to secondary school. Head Start students are monitored informally by the Peer Supporters in Year 7, by the Learning Development team members attached to the Year group and by me as Head Start Programme Leader. Students' performance is also monitored through the school's assessment and tracking system.

The main impact of the programme has been the increased confidence of Year 6 students who were previously anxious about making the transition to secondary school, but who by the end of the programme are really looking forward to coming to secondary school. The programme helps vulnerable students establish and build successful relationships with the Peer Supporters and the other Year 6 students, which leads to much better integration of Head Start students into the school community.

The programme also really helps the school's pastoral team and SEN team to get to know this group of vulnerable students and to plan ahead for their needs in the summer term before they join the school in September. This knowledge informs the composition of tutor groups ensuring the best possible match for vulnerable students with peers and tutors. In the first year of Head Start the school did include a number of students with very extreme behavioural, emotional and social difficulties (BESD) as part of the programme. However, it was felt the programme was not suitable for these students as they tended to form unhelpful groupings with other students with similar problems and they took too much attention away from the other Head Start students. In the following years we have supported these extreme BESD students with more individualized one-to-one support. The impact on Peer Supporters is also significant. In their feedback, Peer Supporters said that they had become more confident in talking to new people and younger children. Importantly, they felt more confident in their communication with children with special needs and more patient and understanding. The programme has had a significant impact on parents and carers. Feedback from parents/carers identifies how they felt reassured about their child's transition to secondary school and this obviously has a large knock-on effect on how their children feel. A further outcome of the programme has been improved relationships and communication with feeder primary schools who really like the programme. These schools now proactively ring the school each year to find out if Head Start is running, as they are already identifying students for the programme even before the referral process starts in summer term.

Here are some evaluations of the Head Start programme:

Year 8 Head Start student

'In Year 6 I was nervous about secondary school. I was worried about the size of the school and I thought I was going to be lost in this really big school and I was scared. I worried about how I would get around the school; would there be places where you could go to do activities? I was worried about leaving behind my friends and about how I would miss all the help they gave me . . . My Peer Supporter really helped; he walked around the school with me and I saw a lot of him in Year 7. My Peer Supporter had similar difficulties with writing and this helped me develop a closer relationship with him.'

Year 7 Head Start student

'When I thought about starting secondary school I was concerned about getting lost in the building, being too shy to say hello to old friends and being too nervous to talk to anyone. Head Start helped because it meant I had two friends (Peer Supporters) who helped me and this made a real difference. I felt less nervous. It also really helped me with understanding the school timetable. The best thing was getting to meet new people, doing completely new things and bringing in a special object to show to other people.'

Head of Year 8

'Head Start has been an invaluable way of cementing our knowledge of the vulnerable Year 6 students transferring to Acland Burghley. The programme enables us to meet the students and interact with them first before we meet the rest of the new Year 7s on induction day. Many of the students come from difficult home situations and their parents and carers are often anxious about establishing communication with the school. The Head Start parent and carer meetings which take place in the evening on one of the Head Start days are attended by all the Year 7 tutors. These meetings provide staff with a bit more time to have personal interactions with parents and carers and this makes a huge difference. The parents and carers feel safer talking to staff and we are able to develop much deeper relationships with them. Through Head Start, the whole process of getting to know students and their families is accelerated by a whole term and staff are able to get a much more holistic picture of each student. Head Start . . . plays an important role in helping us form support networks for students and their families, helping us to sort out the logistics of the support needed and providing a positive foundation on which we can build a programme of interventions to meet each student's needs.'

Head of the Acland Burghley ASD Unit

'There has been a lot of research into the need for slow and repetitive transition for students with ASD. Participation in the Head Start programme has made a huge difference to the ASD student's confidence. They gain a sense of what it will be like being part of their new school. They have the opportunity to know what happens in secondary school and importantly the programme demystifies what it is like to be with older students, making them less scary. I make a point of making sure all the ASD students know beforehand what will be involved in the Head Start programme as launching them into the unknown is very threatening for them and makes them feel very anxious. I go and visit the students beforehand and I explain the timetable of the day and what will be involved in the different activities, thereby reducing the unpredictability of the day. This year, one of the ABC Peer Mentors involved in Head Start was paired with one of the Year 6s with ASD. She has a brother with autism and she worked really well with her student as she was really calm and patient. When the Year 7 induction day came along he met her again and it was really clear that he felt safe with her.'

Discussion questions

Why is it so important for the school to run induction programmes like these for vulnerable students? What are the benefits to school and to the families?

The Head Start team have summarized the key issues that ensure the success of programmes like these in helping vulnerable students build confidence, develop emotional resilience and improve their potential to achieve academically at school:

- Good communication with the primary school. Successful transition takes place where there is good liaison between staff and where information is shared effectively. Primary schools are explicit about the needs of the students. It is important that positive relationships are built between key staff so that primary schools feel they are able to entrust the secondary schools with what is often very sensitive information about their Year 6 students.
- An effective programme should provide opportunities for new students, who are often worried about the large size of secondary schools, to familiarize themselves with the routines and the layout of the secondary school. Getting to know the geography of the school, having access to their Year 7 timetable, understanding how the cafeteria system works and how systems of rewards and sanctions work should all be part of an effective transition programme.
- A good transition programme will seek to reassure the parents and carers of vulnerable students who are also often worried about the unknown. The Head Start programme meetings which provide access for parents and carers to key staff including the head teacher and all the Year 7 tutors have been a key part of the success of the programme.
- You cannot underestimate the central importance of involving older students in any transition programme. As well as the support and friendship they provide they really help to demystify the fears primary students have about older and bigger students.
- Transition is a rite of passage and should be celebrated by the secondary school. It goes without saying that the secondary school should seek to make the experience a positive one and extend a real welcome to the Year 6 students.
- Timing is really important. All schools should hold induction days for students in the summer term. For programmes like Head Start, which seek the more vulnerable students at transition, two weeks before an induction day is about the best time. Students will still

be familiar with the school and they will have a recent contact with peers and Peer Supporters that will improve their experience on the induction day.

Chapter summary

This chapter explores the risk and protective factors that influence the emotional health and well-being of children and young people right from the earliest years. It considers the perspectives of young people, including the stigma that continues to surround the concept of mental health difficulties. This is confirmed by interviews with children and young people who have themselves experienced emotional and behavioural difficulties. There is evidence that young people could offer one another peer support to alleviate at least some of the distress experienced. The chapter distinguishes between internalizing and externalizing disorders. Some effective ways of working with emotionally vulnerable children and young people are described, including one-to-one therapeutic interventions and group work to alleviate potentially distressing events, such as the transition from primary to secondary school. This chapter ends with a case study of one school's strategy for strengthening the resilience of children with social and emotional difficulties as they face the transition from primary to secondary school. It demonstrates the ways in which parents, carers, peers and professionals can collaborate to create systems to facilitate young people's capacity to cope with challenging situations.

Discussion points

- How can adults help protect vulnerable children and young people from the stigma of mental health difficulties?
- How useful is it to distinguish between externalization and internalization in order to understand young people with emotional and behavioural difficulties?
- How can schools create systems to promote emotional health and well-being in children and young people?

Further reading

Cowie, H., Boardman, C., Dawkins, J. & Jennifer, D. (2004) *Emotional Health and Well-being: A Practical Guide for Schools*, London: Sage, provides an accessible overview of practical methods and approaches for supporting children and young people in distress.

Cefai, C. & Cooper, P. (2009) *Promoting Emotional Education*, London: Jessica Kingsley, describes successful humanistic approaches that can be adopted by parents, educators and healthcare professionals to enhance the emotional well-being of all children and young people.

Cairns, E. (1996) *Children and Political Violence*, Oxford: Basil Blackwell, provides important evidence-based information on the impact of war and violence on children's mental health. It also documents children's stress and coping strategies in violent situations.

Boswell, G. (ed.) (2000) *Violent Children and Adolescents: Asking the Question Why*, London: Whurr, explores the reasons that underpin violent behaviour and the strategies that can help to reduce it. See, too: Barter, C. & Berridge, D. (eds) (2011) *Children Behaving Badly*, Chichester: Wiley/Blackwell, for a multidisciplinary perspective on peer violence that explores the issue with regard to, among other aspects, gender, ethnicity, sexuality and poverty.

For research into examination stress, see: Chamberlain, S., Daly, A. & Spalding, V. (2011) 'The fear factor: students' experiences of test anxiety when taking A-level examinations', *Pastoral Care in Education*, 29(3): 193–206.

Websites and resources

YoungMinds is a leading charity committed to improving the emotional health and well-being of children and young people and to empowering their parents and carers:
    http://www.youngminds.org.uk/

The Mental Health Foundation is a charity dedicated to mental health research, policy and service improvement. It campaigns against stigma and helps people of all ages to survive, recover from and prevent mental health problems:
    http://www.mentalhealth.org.uk/

The Royal College of Psychiatrists provides user-friendly information on a wide range of mental health difficulties. The website has a section with useful resources and information for children, young people and for parents and carers:
    http://rcpsych.ac.uk/

See also the 2009 Report from the Children's Commissioner entitled *11 Million: Making Children's Mental Health Matter* on:
    www.11million.org.uk

The European Network for Social and Emotional Competence (ENSEC) is committed to the development of evidence-based practice on the promotion of emotional resilience among school-aged children and young people:
    http://www.enseceurope.org/

Epilogue

Risk and protective factors

The Head Start programme described in Chapter 9 provides one illustration of the ways in which an organization, in this case a school, can provide a nurturing environment for young people who are emotionally vulnerable. What this school is doing in many everyday actions is to strengthen the resilience of the vulnerable children by providing protective factors in their lives to compensate for the risk factors to which they have already been exposed. In the words of Bronfenbrenner (1986: 723), written in the 1980s but even more relevant today:

> At a time of financial entrenchment, when many children are being placed at greater risk as a result of parental unemployment, other income losses, and reduction of health and family services, it is essential to determine which policies and programs can do most to enable families to perform the magic feat of which they alone are capable: making and keeping human beings human.

What Bronfenbrenner refers to here is that prevention and intervention programmes achieve their success by identifying the protective factors that exist within the main systems in which the child or young person is growing up (in this case the school within a community). Subsequently, they strengthen the protective processes (in this case, easing the difficult transition to secondary school by mobilizing the knowledge and experience of specialist staff and trained peer supporters) in order to develop resilience in the vulnerable young people (in this case, acknowledging their understandable fears and anxieties and providing them with enjoyable activities and friendly peers in order to boost their confidence).

The sources of protection in the lives of children and young people can be widened to other challenging areas of experience, as has been indicated throughout this book. As Masten and Garmezy (1985) propose in their influential approach to resilience in the face of adversity, the protective factors operate in three major domains: psychological attributes of the individual; characteristics of the family; characteristics of the social environment. Within this framework, both internal and external factors serve as protective functions for children and adolescents who demonstrate resilience. For example, internal psychological characteristics can shield children from risks, as shown in the study of the resilience shown by some of the vulnerable children in the longitudinal research in Hawaii by Werner and Smith (1982). At the same time, external family and community support can also shield children from at least some of the risks that they currently or previously experienced, for example, the support provided to teenage single mothers by members of the extended family (Borkowski *et al.*, 2007). In each case, protective factors are barriers to risk and so promote the development of resilience. Where researchers and practitioners can collaborate to identify sources of protection in individuals, families and communities, there is greater possibility of helping individuals to develop their own inner resources and, through social and educational support, lessening the negative impact of the difficulties faced by at-risk young people.

Protection within the individual comes from a variety of sources, including gender, self-esteem, intelligence, temperament and **internal locus of control**. High levels of self-esteem as well as pride in achievements, for example, have been shown to protect young people, even those who have faced severe adversity, as indicated in the case study of the English and Romanian adoptees (Chapter 3). Internal locus of control – the perception that the individual has control over the events in his/her life and the capacity to make changes – acts as a powerful buffer against risk factors. Protection within the family, for example, from mothers, fathers, grandparents, can provide a very important source of protection for at-risk children and young people. Parents who prepare their children in the early years for school by engaging in pre-reading activities and developing intersubjectivity through narratives and play, provide a strong buffer against the adversity of poverty and deprivation. Protection from the social environment is also essential, for example, through community networks, neighbourhood projects, membership of churches, by providing positive adult role models and enhancing positive relationships across generations and within peer groups. Clearly, in this context, it is also crucial that there should also be provision of medical care, good schools, housing, social and educational facilities, training and education, job opportunities and good recreational facilities. In other words, protective resources within the child, in the child's family and within the child's social environment are all essential in developing the resilience they need.

For parents, carers and professionals, and all those responsible for the protection and education of children and young people, it is essential to have some understanding of the person in a social and cultural context at a particular point in history. At the time of writing, the nation has been shocked by the outbreak of rioting and looting in city centres, much of it carried out by children and adolescents. Catchphrases abound, such as 'family values have gone' or 'Britain is broken', as do quick-fix solutions, such as 'remove their benefits', 'get the parents to discipline their children', 'bring back respect and authority', 'put the perpetrators in prison'. But these ideas grossly underestimate the complexity of the interplay between the different levels, the contexts in which behaviour happens, the influence of groups, the characteristics of the individuals involved, and the wider social systems that include inequality, disadvantage, exclusion of certain groups, wide variation in access to services and opportunities, and historical events that form part of the collective memory of a nation or social group.

The heart of the child's development lies in the relationships that evolve in myriad everyday ways within the family. Of course, as indicated by Bronfenbrenner's model, there are great differences in the quality of this intimate experience. Throughout, *From Birth to Sixteen* has emphasized the profound influence that attachment relationships have on development in childhood and adolescence. Sensitive attunement on the part of the adult to the child's needs has long-term effects on the child's sense of self, their language development and their capacity to form meaningful relationships with others. At the same time, the individual child or young person also has resources within the self that can be nurtured and fostered to encourage the quality of resilience. Research documents the fact that, despite material disadvantage and emotional neglect, some children grow into happy, secure adolescents and competent adults, indicating that children evolve attachment behaviours as a form of coping in different emotional environments.

Further reading

Smith, H. (1995) *Unhappy Children: Reasons and Remedies*, London: Free Association Books. This book attempts to answer three key questions: What situations might a child encounter while growing up that can lead to a threat to emotional well-being? What emotional needs are not being met? What can be done to help the child to recover a sense of well-being?

Hayden, C. (2007) *Children in Trouble: The Role of Families, Schools and Communities*, Basingstoke: Palgrave Macmillan. This book provides a clear-headed analysis of critical ways in which the nature of adult responses, whether at home, in school or in the community, can impact on the difficulties experienced by troubled children. See too Hayden, C. & Martin, D. (eds) (2011) *Crime, Anti-Social Behaviour and Schools*, Basingstoke: Palgrave Macmillan.

For a critical, multidisciplinary overview of research and practice into peer violence, see: Barter, C. & Berridge, D. (eds) (2011) *Children Behaving Badly*, Chichester: Wiley/Blackwell, as well as Boswell, G. (ed.) (2000) *Violent Children and Adolescents: Asking the Question Why*, London: Whurr.

Websites and resources

The Royal College of Psychiatrists Anti-Stigma Campaign played a substantial part in widening awareness about mental health difficulties and in reducing prejudice. For more information about the campaign see:
    www.iop.kcl.ac.uk

For up-to-date information on young carers and the support that is available for them, see:
    www.carers.org

For information on play therapy see:
    www.playtherapy.org.uk

For information on OCD see:
    www.ocduk.org

and for a helpful guide for young people see the Maudsley Hospital website:
    www.ocdyouth.iop.kcl.ac.uk

For information on stigma see 'See Beyond Our Labels' on the YoungMinds website:
    www.youngminds.org.uk

See also:
    www.ComfortConsults.com

Glossary

Advergaming A marketing practice of using video games to advertise a product, organization or viewpoint. Often used by companies to promote products for children.

Anorexia nervosa An eating disorder involving extreme dietary restriction and various forms of weight control behaviour, such as vomiting, obsessive exercising or laxative misuse, characterized by a refusal to maintain body weight at or above a minimally normal weight for age and height, intense fear of becoming fat, distorted body image and extreme food avoidance.

Anxiety A mental health disorder characterized by overwhelming feelings of unease, fear and uncertainty and by doubt about the reality of the nature of the threatening issue and one's ability to deal with it. Anxiety is often characterized by physical symptoms, such as sweating and tension.

Asperger syndrome A developmental disorder that falls within the broader category of **autistic spectrum disorders** (ASDs). Children and young people with Asperger syndrome demonstrate qualitative impairments in social interaction (e.g., finding it hard to make eye contact), qualitative impairments in communication (e.g., delays in language development, lack of make-believe play) and restrictive or stereotyped patterns of behaviour (e.g., inflexible adherence to routines and rituals, or intense interest in one particular topic, such as astronomy). Individuals with Asperger syndrome find it difficult to develop a **theory of mind**. In other words, they have problems in understanding that other people have independent beliefs and often find it difficult to understand why others behave as they do.

Attachment theory John Bowlby's lifelong work on attachment theory began shortly after he graduated when he worked in a residential home for maladjusted boys. He observed the intense distress experienced by these children when separated from their mothers, even when they were fed and cared for by others. He became convinced that major disruptions in the mother-child relationship are the precursors of later psychopathology. Bowlby (1969) proposed that the child uses the mother, or primary caregiver, as a secure base to return to regularly for reassurance, and identified the following phases in the development of attachment: in the first few months of life, the infant does not discriminate between different people; later, usually around 5–7 months of age, the infant preferentially orientates to one or two significant adults, usually the parents; from 7–9 months of age begins the onset of attachment when the infant becomes wary of strangers; from 2–3 years of age, the child develops a goal-directed partnership that accommodates to the parent/caregiver's needs; by school age, the child is developing a more abstract concept of attachment – the **internal working model of relationships** – based on affection, trust and approval.

Autistic spectrum disorder (ASD) ASDs begin in childhood and persist throughout adolescence and adulthood. There are a wide range of symptoms which can broadly be categorized as: i) difficulties with social interaction and a lack of awareness of other people's emotions and feelings; ii) impaired language and communication skills; iii) unusual patterns of thought and behaviour, including repetitive physical movements and set routines of behaviour.

Body Mass Index (BMI) The most common measure of weight status, calculated by weight in kilograms divided by the square of height in metres.

Bulimia nervosa An eating disorder involving various forms of weight control behaviour, such as vomiting, obsessive exercising or laxative misuse, binges followed by vomiting, excessive fasting or exercising.

Cognitive Behavioural Therapy (CBT) A form of psychotherapy involving the client in examining the links between thoughts, feelings and behaviour. CBT helps the client to manage problems by changing the ways in which they think and act in order to find practical ways of dealing with their problems. Unlike many other talking therapies, CBT focuses on the present rather than on emotional issues from the past. It is very effective in dealing with **anxiety, depression**, eating disorders and drug misuse.

Co-morbidity The presence of more than one major health disorder in an individual.

Creole language This is a language that was originally a **pidgin** but which, over time, became the first language of a community of speakers. In contrast to pidgin languages, Creole languages have a grammatical structure. The term Creole has been used to designate the language of people of Caribbean and African descent in colonial or ex-colonial countries, such as Jamaica, Haiti and Hawaii.

Depression One of the commonest mental health disorders in children and young people. Typical aspects include persistent feelings of sadness, inability to concentrate, apathy, withdrawal from social interaction, low self-esteem and suicidal ideation.

Egocentric empathic distress The child's response to a distressing situation that indicates difficulty in distinguishing between the distress of another and their own distress.

Egocentric speech According to Vygotsky, between the ages of 2 and 7 years language serves two main functions: i) the monitoring and direction of internal thoughts; and ii) the communication of these thoughts to others. The young child cannot yet distinguish between these internal and external functions and so will often engage thinking aloud, or egocentric speech, about ongoing plans and actions. The function of egocentric speech is closely connected with the child's thinking processes.

Emotional intelligence (EI) Salovey and Mayer (1990) identified five core EI abilities: the capacity to understand feelings of self and others; the capacity to manage feelings and to help others to manage their feelings; self-motivation and the capacity for delayed gratification of emotional needs; the ability to handle relationships; the development of empathy in order to build on emotional self-awareness. There is controversy in the field about how to measure EI. Petrides and Furnham (2001) distinguish between the concept of EI as an ability and EI as a subjective emotional experience.

Emotional literacy A pedagogical approach designed to enhance emotional intelligence by developing a child-centred teaching style and a supportive learning community in the classroom. Bruce (2010) defines emotional literacy as a way of *being* rather than of *doing*. The teacher's role is to provide a safe but challenging learning environment where children are free to grow socially and emotionally.

Empathic distress When people observe another person in distress, they typically respond empathically (that is, with feelings that are more congruent with that other person's feelings than with their own) or with a helpful action. Hoffman (2000) views empathic distress as a prosocial motive that precedes helpful behaviour, contributes to helpful behaviour, diminishes when one offers help and stays at a high level when one does not help.

Empathy The capacity to relate to the thoughts, emotions and experiences of another person. Hoffman (2000: 29–30) indicates that empathy has been defined in two ways: i) as the cognitive awareness of another person's internal states; or ii) as the vicarious affective response to another person. He prefers the latter and defines empathy in terms of 'the involvement of psychological processes that make a person have feelings that are more congruent with another's situation than with his own situation. Empathy is closely related to the development of the child's concept of self and eventually to the development of such concepts as caring and justice.'

Externalizing emotional difficulties The process of acting out emotional difficulties, for example, through conduct disorders, by taking drugs and alcohol excessively or engaging in disruptive behaviour.

Holophrase A single word used to express a complete thought. The term is used to describe the utterances of children in which a single word expresses the meaning that in adult speech would usually be conveyed in a whole sentence. For example, 'Milk!' can mean 'I want more milk!'

Ideal self The self that the person would ideally like to be. The greater the gap between self-image and ideal self, the lower the person's **self-esteem** is likely to be.

Identity achievement One of the four states proposed by Marcia (1993) in the process of identity formation during adolescence. In this state, the young person emerges from the struggle to form an identity with clear commitments, goals, values and aspirations.

Identity diffusion One of the four states proposed by Marcia (1993) in the process of identity formation during adolescence. In this state, the young person is in crisis and finds it difficult to achieve a clear sense of **self-concept**.

Identity foreclosure One of the four states proposed by Marcia (1993) in the process of identity formation during adolescence. In this state, the young person avoids the uncertainty and anxiety of crisis by committing themselves to safe, conventional goals without exploring the many options open to them.

Identity moratorium One of the four states proposed by Marcia (1993) in the process of identity formation during adolescence. In this state, the young person postpones making decisions about their identity and experiments with a range of roles. They might, for example, experiment with different sexual and romantic partners. They might rebel against adult values by identifying with rebellious groups. They might dress in provocative, challenging ways.

Inner speech Inner speech represents a central process in consciousness, memory and thinking, emerging as **egocentric speech** in younger children and then later as self-directed, inner speech in older children through adolescence to adulthood. It plays a primary role in the regulation of thought and behaviour and features in such activities as reading, writing, speaking and doing mathematical calculations.

Internal locus of control An individual's perception that they have control over the events in their life and the capacity to make changes. It is a powerful protective factor against low **self-esteem**.

Internal working model of relationships (IWM) The IWM is a set of memories and cognitions based on experiences of the relationship with the primary caregivers (usually parents) that guide the child's actions and emotions. Children develop the ability to think about attachment relationships even when the primary caregiver is not present. The IWM is a cognitive structure that embodies the memories of day-to-day interactions with the primary caregiver. These event scripts guide the child's actions and expectations with regard to the attachment figure, based on previous interactions. The child is forming a sense of intimate relationships that does not only rely on physical proximity but on qualities, such as affection, trust and feelings of being valued.

Internalizing mental health difficulties The process of turning emotional difficulties inwards and so being more likely to become depressed, fearful or anxious.

Intersubjectivity The process through which children and adults communicate, regulate and maintain their interactions with one another. It refers to shared meanings and cognitions and is at the heart of the development of ideas and relationships.

Language acquisition device (LAD) This is a hypothetical explanatory model proposed by Chomsky (1965) to explain language development. It is based on the assumption that individuals are born with the propensity to understand the rules that transform the deep structure of language into the surface structures of their own particular language. Chomsky argued that certain features of language were universal, that is, common to all languages. Only the concept of LAD could explain the rapidity with which children learn to speak grammatically, no matter which language they are exposed to.

Makaton A language programme using signs and symbols to help people with learning disabilities or communication difficulties. It is designed to support spoken language and the signs and symbols are used with speech in spoken word order.

Mind-mindedness This refers to the adult's ability or willingness to represent their children's thoughts and feelings. It is the way that a parent or carer treats their infant as an individual with a mind rather than simply as a creature with needs to be met. Maternal mind-mindedness is related to some key developmental outcomes, such as security of attachment and **theory of mind**. Mind-mindedness on the part of adult carers is important from the very earliest years of the child's life, and can be expressed, for example, through language and playful interactions.

Narcissism/false self-esteem The tendency to hold favourable self-appraisals that may not be grounded in reality or may be exaggerated; often includes difficulty in accepting any form of criticism. Narcissistic individuals are preoccupied with themselves, need to seek out attention, and have a heightened concern to win the approval of others that they consider to be important.

Nurture groups (NGs) The practice of NGs is grounded in **attachment theory** and is a teaching method that aims to compensate for the emotional and social difficulties experienced by some children in forming trusting, positive relationships with peers, siblings and adults. The NG teacher's role is to understand the gaps in the children's experiences at home and to try to meet their particular needs. Typically, the children spend most of the school week in the NG, a small group of usually no more than eight children, gradually joining in mainstream classes as they become emotionally ready.

Obesity Excessive weight in relation to age or height, usually measured by the **Body Mass Index** (BMI).

Object permanence Very young babies will look at an object and follow it with their eyes, but as soon as it goes out of sight, they make no attempt to look for it, as if it no longer existed. By around 8 months of age, the baby will search for an object that has been hidden. In other words, the baby now appears to have a sense that the object exists independently. The baby has now developed object permanence.

Obsessive compulsive disorder (OCD) OCD is an anxiety disorder characterized by obsessive thoughts, compulsive behaviours and repetitive rituals that interfere with normal daily life. For example, a person may be so obsessed with thoughts about germs that they feel compelled to wash repeatedly in order to be clean. The most effective treatment for OCD is **Cognitive Behavioural Therapy** (CBT) which teaches healthy, constructive ways of responding to obsessive thoughts and of dealing with compulsive behaviour.

Person permanence Person permanence usually begins to develop between 8 and 12 months of age, with major progress towards the end of the first year. It has been assessed in terms of infants' recognition of particular others, and the search for them when that person disappears from view. Person permanence implies the internal representation of a social being, corresponding to that person's continuity in time. It is closely related to **object permanence**. At this stage, the infant appears to understand that other people have a separate and permanent existence, even when not in sight.

Pidgin language This type of language arises when two or more people who do not share a common language need to communicate, for example, for purposes of work, often in conditions of slavery or colonialism. Pidgins are a mixture of these languages. Typically, they do not have consistent word order, tenses or any structures more complex than simple clauses. The prestige of pidgin languages is usually very low.

Pivot grammar Used by children at a particular stage of their language development at around 18 months of age when they have only a limited range of pivot words that they use in conjunction with other words in order to convey meaning. One example is 'more' in conjunction with things that the child wants, for example, 'more milk', 'more biscuit'. Pivot grammar evolves as the young child develops a greater understanding of the concept of more complex grammatical structures.

Runaways Children or young people who run away from home without parental permission.

Self-concept Self and self-concept are often used interchangeably to refer to the individual's self-awareness. There are three interrelated aspects: **self-image, self-esteem** and **ideal self**.

Self-esteem In contrast to **self-image**, which is descriptive, self-esteem is the person's evaluation of the self, and refers to the extent to which the self is valued by that person. Self-esteem is strongly influenced by the person's social context and by the values held by members of the person's social group.

Self-image The descriptive way in which a person portrays or represents themselves, often in terms of social identity, personal appearance or personality. For example, gender is one core aspect of self-image. The person's self-image can be elicited by asking for repeated responses to the question 'Who am I?'

Separation anxiety In children, this is a form of anxiety expressed by excessive clinging to parents and acute anxiety about being separated from them, for example, when the child is required to attend school.

Sexually abusive behaviour Sexual behaviour initiated by a person where there is use of manipulation or force, or where the target is unable to give informed consent.

Sexually problematic behaviour Sexual activity that may interfere with the child's development or increase that child's risk of rejection or victimization.

Social story books Books designed for children and young people who find it hard to develop a **theory of mind**. The books feature stories and cartoons with information on what the characters are doing, thinking or feeling, sequences of typical social events, identification of significant social happenings, and scripts on what to say and do in these situations. They also make use of **thought bubbles** to convey information on what characters are thinking and feeling in different situations.

Sociometric status Children's sociometric status – or their position in the structure of peer relationships – can be inferred in the following ways: by direct observation of their behaviour with peers; by asking an adult, such as a parent or teacher; or by asking children about their friendship choices. Through these methods, it is possible to build up a picture of how children interact with one another, which children are frequently chosen by peers, which are rejected or ignored, which spend most time with one special friend, whether or not boys and girls interact with one another. One common method for identifying sociometric status is to ask each child in a class to name their three best friends. Children can then be categorized on the basis of these choices. The most common types elicited by the method are: average, popular, controversial, rejected and neglected. Children who are rejected or neglected by peers have a more stressful experience of social interaction and are more likely to continue to have relationship difficulties throughout childhood. Average children typically have one or two friends with whom they spend a great deal of time. Popular children are chosen by many of their peers as friends. Controversial children are both admired and feared by peers on the basis of their power and aggressiveness.

Symbolic interactionism The theory proposed by George Herbert Mead (1934) that there is a distinction between the 'I' (self as knower) and the 'me' (self as known). Mead proposed a reflexive process through which we stand back from the self in order to interact with it and experience it. The symbolic interactionist position states that the self-concept evolves when the child takes the perspective of significant others in his/her life and so comes to see the self as an object as seen through the eyes of others.

Theory of mind/mind-reading The ability to hypothesize about what is going on in another's mind; the capacity to attribute mental states, such as emotions, desires and beliefs, to the self as well as to others. From about 2 years of age, children will start to use words that refer to internal states of perception or emotion, but they do not achieve theory of mind fully until around 4 years of age. The child's theory of mind can be assessed through false-belief tasks (e.g., the Ellie the Elephant Coke test) which test the child's capacity to infer what another is thinking by taking that person's point of view rather than their own. There is some evidence that children who have wide experience of talking extensively with siblings, peers and adults about experiences and emotions will be successful on theory of mind tasks at an earlier age.

Thought bubbles These are cartoons used in **social story books** with thought bubbles coming out of the characters' heads to portray what they are thinking in different social situations. The teaching method is used to help children with **Asperger syndrome** to develop techniques for dealing with a range of social situations that they often find difficult.

Universal grammar Chomsky's (1965) theory proposes that all languages have universal properties, including phonological aspects such as consonants, vowels and syllables and a grammatical structure. According to this theory, all humans have an innate **language acquisition device** (LAD) without which language could not develop.

Verb-island hypothesis Developed by Michael Tomasello to propose that children's early grammar development consists of sets of specific structures or verb islands. Verbs do not operate as a coherent class but as individual 'islands' of organization. In other words, children acquire the combinatorial rules of grammar verb by verb.

Young carers Children or young people who are responsible for caring for an adult in their family who is ill.

Bibliography

Abdunnur, S. & Hartley, J. S. (2007) *Laughter Under the Bombs: Diaries of a Dramatherapist*. Milton Keynes: Author House UK Ltd.

Aboud, F. (1988) *Children and Prejudice*. Oxford: Basil Blackwell.

Adams, M. J. (1990) *Beginning to Read: Thinking and Learning About Print*. Cambridge, MA: MIT Press.

Ainsworth, M. D. S. (1967) *Infancy in Uganda: Infant Care and the Growth of Attachment*. Baltimore, MD: Johns Hopkins University Press.

Ainsworth, M. D. S., Blehar, M., Waters, E. & Wall, S. (1978) *Patterns of Attachment: A Psychological Study of the Strange Situation*. Hillsdale, NJ: Lawrence Erlbaum.

Alcohol Concern (2010) *Right Time, Right Place*. London: Alcohol Concern.

Aldrich, N. J., Tenenbaum, H. R., Brooks, P. J., Harrison, K. & Sines, J. (2011) 'Perspective taking in children's narratives about jealousy', *British Journal of Developmental Psychology*, 29(1): 86–109.

Aldridge, J., Measham, F. & Williams, L. (2011) *Illegal Leisure Revisited*. London: Routledge.

Ali, M., Blades, M., Oates, C. & Blumberg, F. (2009) 'Children's ability to recognize advertisements on Web pages', *British Journal of Developmental Psychology*, 27: 71–84.

American Academy of Pediatrics Committee on Public Education (2001) 'Children, adolescents and television', *Pediatrics*, 117(2): 423–426.

American Psychological Association (2004) *Report of the APA Task Force on Advertising and Children*. Accessed August 2011 from www.apa.org

Anderson, C. A., Sakamoto, A., Gentile, D., Ihori, N., Shibuya, A., Yukawa, S., Naito, M. & Kobayashi, K. (2008) 'Longitudinal effects of violent video games on aggression in Japan and the United States', *Pediatrics*, 122(5): e1067–e1072.

Anderson, C. A., Shibuya, A., Ihori, N., Swing, E. L., Bushman, B. J., Sakamoto, A., Rothstein, H. R. & Saleem, M. (2010) 'Violent video game effects on aggression, empathy, and prosocial behavior in Eastern and Western countries: a meta-analytic review', *Psychological Bulletin*, 136: 151–173.

Armstrong, C., Hill, H. & Secker, J. (2000) 'Young people's perceptions of mental health', *Children and Society*, 14: 60–72.

Arnold, C., Yeomans, J. & Simpson, S. (2009) *Excluded from School*. Stoke-on-Trent: Trentham Books.

Asthana, A. (2007) 'Imaginary pals: a tonic for children', *The Observer*, 8 July, News section: 20.

Aylett, R. S., Louchart, S., Dias, J., Paiva, A. & Vala, M. (2005) 'FearNot!: an experiment in emergent narrative', in T. Panayiotopoulos, J. Gratch, R. Aylett, D. Ballin, P. Olivier & T. Rist (eds) *Proceedings of Intelligent Virtual Agents (IVA) 2005 Conference*. Hamburg: Springer, pp. 305–316.

Aynsley-Green, A. (2009) *11 Million: Making Children's Mental Health Matter*. London: Office of the Children's Commissioner. Accessed August 2011 from www.11million.org.uk

Bacon, L. (2008) *Health at Every Size: The Surprising Truth About Your Weight*. Dallas, TX: BenBella Books.

Bacon, L., Van Loon, M., Stern, J. S. & Keim, N. (2005) 'Size acceptance and intuitive eating improve health for obese, female chronic dieters' (abstract page), *Journal of the American Dietetic Association*, 105(6): 929–936.

Balbernie, R. & Gorney, C. (2011) 'Unlocking the potential', *YoungMinds Magazine*, 110: 22–23.

Baldry, A. & Farrington, D. P. (2007) 'Effectiveness of programmes to prevent school bullying', *Victims and Offenders*, 2: 183–204.

Banerjee, R. (2010) *Social and Emotional Aspects of Learning in Schools: A Report on Data from the National Strategies, Tracker School Project*. University of Sussex. Accessed July 2011 from http://nationalstrategies.standards.dcsf.gov.uk/node/486406

Barnardo's (2007) *It Doesn't Happen Here: The Reality of Child Poverty in the UK*. London: Barnardo's.

Barnes, K. (2003) 'Behavioural problems and inappropriate sexual behaviour', in K. Barnes (ed.) *Paediatrics: A Clinical Guide for Nurse Practitioners*. Oxford: Butterworth-Heinemann, pp. 189–212.

Baron-Cohen, S., Tager-Flusberg, H. & Cohen, D. J. (2000) 'A note on nosology', in S. Baron-Cohen, H. Tager-Flusberg & D. J. Cohen (eds) *Understanding Other Minds: Perspectives from Developmental Cognitive Neuroscience*. Oxford: Oxford University Press.

Barrett, M. (2007) *Children's Knowledge, Beliefs and Feelings about Nations and National Groups*. Hove: Psychology Press.

Barrett, M. & Oppenheimer, L. (2011) 'Findings, theories and methods in the study of children's national identifications and national attitudes', *European Journal of Developmental Psychology*, 8: 1, 5–24.

Barrett, M., Wilson, H. & Lyons, E. (2003) 'The development of national in-group bias: English children's attributions of characteristics to English, American and German people', *British Journal of Developmental Psychology*, 21: 193–220.

Barter, C. (2009) 'In the name of love: exploitation and violence in teenage dating relationships', *British Journal of Social Work*, 39: 211–233.

Barter, C. (2011) 'A thoroughly gendered affair: teenage partner violence and exploitation', in C. Barter & D. Berridge (eds) *Children Behaving Badly: Peer Violence Between Children and Young People*. Chichester: Wiley/Blackwell, pp. 103–120.

Barter, C. & Berridge, D. (2011) *Children Behaving Badly: Peer Violence Between Children and Young People*. Chichester: Wiley/Blackwell.

Barter, C., McCarry, M., Berridge, D. & Evans, K. (2009) *Partner Exploitation and Violence in Teenage Intimate Relationships*. London: National Society for the Prevention of Cruelty to Children.

Bauermeister, J., Johns, M. M., Sandfort, T. G., Eiosenberg, A., Grossman, A. H. & D'Augelli, A. R. (2010) 'Relationship trajectories and psychological well-being among sexual minority youth', *Journal of Youth and Adolescence*, 39: 1148–1163.

Baumeister, R. F. (2001) 'Violent pride', *Scientific American*, 284(4): 96–101.

Baumeister, R. F., Smart, L. & Boden, J. M. (1996) 'Relation of threatened egotism to violence and aggression: the dark side of high self-esteem', *Psychological Review*, 103: 5–33.

Bibliography

Begley, A. (1999) 'The self-perceptions of pupils with Down syndrome in relation to their academic competence, physical competence and social acceptance', *International Journal of Disability, Development and Education*, 46: 515–529.

Beinart, S., Anderson, B., Lee, S. & Utting, D. (2002) *Youth at Risk? A National Survey of Risk Factors, Protective Factors and Problem Behaviour Among Young People in England, Scotland and Wales*. London: Communities that Care.

Belsky, J. (2006) 'Effects of child care on child development in the USA', in J. J. van Kuyk (ed.) *The Quality of Early Childhood Education*. Arnheim, The Netherlands: Cito, pp. 23–32.

Belsky, J. (2010) 'Do effects of early child care extend to age 15 years? Results from the NICHD study of early child care and youth development', *Child Development*, 8(3): 737–756.

Belsky, J. & Melhuish, E. (2007) 'Impact of Sure Start local programmes on children and families', in J. Belsky, J. Barnes & E. Melhuish (eds) (2007) *The National Evaluation of Sure Start*. Bristol: The Policy Press, pp. 133–153.

Belsky, J. & Melhuish, E. (2008) *The Impact of Sure Start Local Programmes on Three-Year-Olds and Their Families*. London: DfES.

Bennathan, M. & Boxall, M. (1998) *The Boxall Profile: A Guide to Effective Intervention in the Education of Pupils with Emotional and Behavioural Difficulties*. Maidstone: AWCEBD.

Bennett, M., Barrett, M., Karakozov, R., Kipiani, G., Lyons, E., Pavlenko, V. & Riazanova, T. (2004) 'Young children's evaluations of the ingroup and of outgroups: a multi-national study', *Social Development*, 13: 124–141.

Bickerton, D. (1990) *Language and Species*. Chicago, IL: University of Chicago Press.

Borkowski, J. G., Farris, J. R., Whitman, T. L., Carothers, S. S., Weed, K. & Keogh, D. A. (2007) *Risk and Resilience: Adolescent Mothers and their Children Grow Up*. Mahwah, NJ: Lawrence Erlbaum.

Bowlby, J. (1969) *Attachment and Loss. Volume 1*. London: Hogarth Press.

Bowlby, J. (1988) *A Secure Base*. New York: Basic Books.

Bronfenbrenner, U. (1979) *The Ecology of Human Development*. Cambridge, MA: Harvard University Press.

Bronfenbrenner, U. (1986) 'Ecology of the family as a context for human development: research perspectives', *Developmental Psychology*, 22: 723–774.

Brown, B. B. (1999) '"You're going out with who?" Peer group influences on adolescent romantic relationships', in W. Furman, B. B. Brown & C. Feiring (eds) *The Development of Romantic Relationships in Adolescence*. New York: Cambridge University Press, pp. 291–329.

Brown, J. R., Donelan-McCall, N. & Dunn, J. (1996) 'Why talk about mental states? The significance of children's conversations with friends, siblings, and mothers', *Child Development*, 67: 836–849.

Brown, R. A. J. & Renshaw, P. (2000) 'Collective argumentation: a sociocultural approach to reframing classroom teaching and learning', in H. Cowie & G. van der Aalsvoort (eds) *Social Interaction in Learning and Instruction*. Amsterdam: Elsevier Science, pp. 52–66.

Bruce, C. (2010) *Emotional Literacy in the Early Years*. London: Sage.

Bryan, K. (ed.) (2009) *Communication in Healthcare*. Bern: Peter Lang.

Bryant, P. E. & Bradley, L. (1986) *Children's Reading Problems*. Oxford: Basil Blackwell.

Bryant, P. E., MacLean, M., Bradley, L. L. & Crossland, J. (1990) 'Rhyme and alliteration, phoneme detection, and learning to read', *Developmental Psychology*, 26(3): 429–438.

Burgoyne, K. (2009) 'The link between gesture and speech in children with Down syndrome', *Down Syndrome Research and Practice*, 12(3): 173–174.

Bushman, B. J. & Baumeister, R. F. (1998) 'Threatened egotism, narcissism, self-esteem and direct and displaced aggression: does self-love or self-hate lead to violence?', *Journal of Personality and Social Psychology*, 75: 219–229.

Byron, T. (2008) *Safer Children in Digital World: The Report of the Byron Review*. Accessed 1 November 2010 from http://www.dcsf.gov.uk/byronreview/

Calamaro, C. J. & Waite, R. (2009) 'Depression and obesity in adolescence: what can primary providers do?', *The Journal for Nurse Practitioners*, 5(4): 255–261.

Card, N. A. (2010) 'Antipathetic relationships in child and adolescent development: a meta-analytic review and recommendations for an emerging area of study', *Developmental Psychology*, 46: 516–529.

Cassidy, J. (1999) 'The nature of a child's ties', in J. Cassidy & P. R. Shaver (eds) *Handbook of Attachment*. New York: Guilford Press, pp. 3–20.

Cater, S. & Coleman, J. (2006) *'Planned' Teenage Pregnancy: Perspectives of Young Parents from Disadvantaged Backgrounds*. Bristol: The Policy Press.

Cater, S. & McDowell, A. (2010) *Pregnancy Rates, Attitudes and Behaviour Changes Among Graduates of Teens and Toddlers: Annual Retrospective Study 2008*. London: Teens and Toddlers Project. Accessed August 2011 from www.teensandtoddlers.org.uk

Cattanach, A. (1994) *Play Therapy: Where the Sky Meets the Underworld*. London: Jessica Kingsley.

Cefai, C. & Cooper, P. (2009) *Promoting Emotional Education*. London: Jessica Kingsley.

Chaffinch, M., Berliner, L., Block, R., Cavanagh Johnson, T., Friedrich, W. N., Garcia Louis, D., Lyon, T. D., Page, I. J., Prescott, D. S., Silkovsky, J. F. & Madden, C. (2008) 'Report of the Association for the Treatment of Sexual Abusers (ATSA) Task Force on children with sexual behaviour problems', *Child Maltreatment*, 13(2): 199–218.

Chamberlain, S., Daly, A. & Spalding, V. (2011) 'The fear factor: students' experiences of test anxiety when taking A-level examinations', *Pastoral Care in Education*, 29(3): 193–206.

Children's Society, The (2011) *Make Runaways Safe*. London: The Children's Society.

Chomsky, N. (1965) *Aspects of a Theory of Syntax*. Cambridge, MA: MIT Press.

Chomsky, N. (1986) *Knowledge of Language*. New York: Praeger.

Clarke-Stewart, K. (1989) 'Infant day care: maligned or malignant?', *American Psychologist*, 44: 266–273.

Clay, M. M. (1985) *The Early Detection of Reading Difficulties: A Diagnostic Survey with Recovery Procedures*, 3rd edition. Auckland: Heinemann.

Coleman, J. & Brooks, F. (2009) *Key Data on Adolescence*. Brighton: Young People in Focus, www.youngpeopleinfocus.org.uk

Comfort Consults. Accessed August 2011 from www.ComfortConsults.com

Conners, F. A., Rosenquist, C. J., Arnett, L., Moore, M. S. & Hume, L. E. (2008) 'Improving memory span in children with Down syndrome', *Journal of Intellectual Disability Research*, 52(3): 244–255.

Cooper, P. & Whitebread, D. (2007) 'The effectiveness of Nurture Groups on student progress: evidence from a national research study', *Emotional and Behavioural Difficulties*, 12(3): 171–190.

Cooper, P., Arnold, R. & Boyd, E. (2001) 'The effectiveness of Nurture Groups: preliminary research findings', *British Journal of Special Education*, 28(4): 160–166.

Cowie, H. (2002) 'Not bystanding but standing by: strategies for pupils to cope with bullying', *New Era in Education*, 83(2): 41–43.

Cowie, H. & Jennifer, D. (2008) *New Perspectives on Bullying*. Maidenhead: Open University Press.

Cowie, H. & Olafsson, R. (2000) 'The role of peer support in helping the victims of bullying in a school with high levels of aggression', *School Psychology International*, 21(79): 79–95.

Cowie, H. & Smith, P. K. (2010) 'Peer support as a means of improving school safety and reducing school bullying and violence', in B. Doll, W. Pfohl & J. Yoon (eds) *Handbook of Youth Prevention Science*. New York: Routledge, pp. 177–193.

Cowie, H., Boardman, C., Dawkins, J. & Jennifer, D. (2004) *Emotional Health and Wellbeing: A Practical Guide for Schools*. London: Sage.

Cremin, H., Harrison, T., Mason, C. & Warwick, P. (2011) *Engaging Practice*. University of Cambridge/University of Leicester. Accessed August 2011 from www.engaged.educ.ac.uk

Crittenden, P. M. (1988) 'Relationships as risk', in J. Belsky & T. Nezworski (eds) *Clinical Implications of Attachment*. Hillsdale, NJ: Lawrence Erlbaum, pp. 136–174.

Crittenden, P. M. (1992) 'The quality of attachment in the preschool years', *Development and Psychopathology*, 4: 209–241.

Crittenden, P. M. (1995) 'Attachment and psychopathology', in S. Goldberg, R. Muir & J. Kerr (eds) *Attachment Theory: Social Developmental and Clinical Perspectives*. Hillsdale, NJ: Analytic Press, pp. 367–406.

Currie, C. (2010) *Message in a Bottle: A Joint Inspection of Youth Alcohol Misuse and Offending*. Accessed August 2011 from www.cqc.org.uk/_db/_documents/Inspecting_ Youth_Offending_Thematic_-_Alcohol_Misuse_

Currie, C., Roberts, C. & Morgan, A. (2008) *Health Behaviour in School-aged Children. International Report from the 2005/2006 Study*. Geneva: World Health Organization.

Daly, A. L. (2006) 'Bullying, victimisation, self-esteem, and narcissism in adolescents'. Unpublished Ph.D. thesis, Flinders University School of Education, South Australia.

Darwin, C. (1877) 'A biological sketch of an infant', *Mind: Quarterly Review of Psychology and Philosophy*, 11: 286–294.

Davila, J., Steinberg, S. J., Kachadourian, L., Cobb, R. & Fincham, F. (2004) 'Romantic involvement and depressive symptoms in early and late adolescence: the role of a preoccupied relational style', *Personal Relationships*, 11(2): 161–178.

Department for Children, Schools and Families (DCSF) (2005) *Excellence and Enjoyment: Social and Emotional Aspects of Learning*. Norwich: HMSO.

Department for Children, Schools and Families (DCSF) (2007) *Social and Emotional Aspects of Learning for Secondary Schools*. Nottingham: HMSO.

Department for Children, Schools and Families (DCSF) (2008) *Targeted Mental Health in Schools Programme: Every Child Matters*. Nottingham: HMSO.

Department of Health (DH) (2004) *Choosing Health: Making Healthy Choices Easier*. London: HMSO.

Department of Health (DH) (2010) *Healthy Lives, Healthy People: Our Strategy for Public Health in England*. London: HMSO. Accessed August 2011 from http://www.dh.gov.uk/en/ Publichealth/Healthyliveshealthypeople/index.htm

Department of Health/Department of Education (2009) *Healthy Lives, Brighter Futures: The Strategy for Young People's Health*. London: HMSO.

Dissanayake, E. (2000) 'Antecedents of the temporal arts in early mother-infant interaction', in N. L. Wallin, B. Merker & S. Brown (eds) *The Origin of the Mind*. Cambridge, MA: MIT Press, pp. 389–410.

Doak, C. M., Visscher, T. L. S., Renders, C. M. & Seidell, J. C. (2006) 'The prevention of overweight and obesity in children and adolescents', *Obesity Reviews*, 7: 111–136.

Donaldson, L. (2009) *Draft Guidance on the Consumption of Alcohol by Children and Young People: A Report by the Chief Medical Officer*. London: Department of Health. Accessed April 2011 from http://www.dh.gov.uk/

Doutre, G. & Mansfield, D. (2010) 'Food for thought: children's views on the psychological aspects of childhood obesity'. Unpublished doctoral thesis, University of Bristol.

Dunn, J., Brown, J. & Beardsall, L. (1991) 'Family talk about feeling states and children's later understanding of others' emotions', *Developmental Psychology*, 27: 448–455.

Dyregrov, A. (1990) *Grief in Children*. London: Jessica Kingsley.

Erikson, E. (1968) *Identity, Youth and Crisis*. New York: Norton.

Eron, L. D. (1987) 'The development of aggressive behavior from the perspective of a developing behaviorism', *American Psychologist*, 42: 435–442.

Escobar, M., Fernandez-Baen, F. J., Miranda, J., Trianes, M. V. & Cowie, H. (2011) 'Low peer acceptance and emotional/behavioural maladjustment in schoolchildren: effects of daily stress, coping and sex', *Anales de Psicologia*, 27(2): 412–417.

Eskin, M. (1995) 'Adolescents' attitudes towards suicide and a suicidal peer: a comparison between Swedish and Turkish high school students', *Scandinavian Journal of Psychology*, 36(2): 201–207.

Evans Schmidt, M., Bickham, D. S., Branner, A. & Rich, M. (2008) 'Media related policies of professional health organizations', in S. L. Calvert & B. J. Wilson (eds) *The Handbook of Children, Media and Development*. Oxford: Basil Blackwell.

Farrington, D. P. (1995) 'The twelfth Jack Tizard memorial lecture: the development of offending and antisocial behaviour from childhood: key findings from the Cambridge Study in Delinquent Development', *Journal of Child Psychology and Psychiatry*, 36(6): 929–964.

Farrington, D. P. & Baldry, A. (2010) 'Individual risk factors for school bullying', *Journal of Aggression, Conflict and Peace Research*, 2: 4–16.

Fearn, M. & Howard, J. (2012, in press) 'Play as a resource for children facing adversity: an exploration of indicative case studies', *Children & Society*.

Fernyhough, C. (2008) *The Baby in the Mirror: A Child's World from Birth to Three*. London: Granta.

Field-Smith, M. E., Bland, J. M., Taylor, J. C., Ramsey, J. D. & Anderson, H. R. (2002) 'Trends in death associated with abuse of volatile substances', London: St George's Hospital Medical School. Accessed August 2011 from www.sghms.ac.uk/depts/phs/vsa2000

Fogel, A. (1993) 'Two principles of communication: co-regulation and framing', in J. Nadel & L. Camaioni (eds) *New Perspectives in Early Communication Development*. London: Routledge, pp. 9–22.

Fonagy, P., Steele, H. & Steele, M. (1991) 'Maternal representations of attachment during pregnancy predict the organisation of infant-mother attachment at one year of age', *Child Development*, 62: 891–905.

Fonagy, P., Steele, H., Steele, M. & Holder, J. (1997) 'Attachment and theory of mind: overlapping constructs?', Association of Child Psychology and Psychiatry Occasional Papers No. 14, *Bonding and Attachment*: 31–40.

Frances, G. (2010) *Teenage Pregnancy: Part Successes, Future Challenges*, Teenage Pregnancy Advisory Group (TPIAG) Final report. London: TPIAG, Teenage Pregnancy Unit, DfE, Great Smith Street, London SW1P 3BT.

Gale, E. & Holling, A. (2000) 'Young people and stigma', *YoungMinds Magazine*: 49–50.

Goleman, D. (1995) *Emotional Intelligence*. London: Bloomsbury.

Goodman, R. (1997) 'The strengths and difficulties questionnaire: a research note', *Journal of Child Psychology and Psychiatry*, 38(5): 581–586.

Goswami, U. (1995) 'Phonological development and reading by analogy: what is analogy and what is not?', *Journal of Research in Reading*, 18(2): 139–145.

Gracey, D., Stanley, N., Burke, V., Corti, B. & Bellin, L. J. (1996) 'Nutritional knowledge, beliefs and behaviours in teenager school students', *Health Education Research*, 11: 187–204.

Gray, A., Pithers, W. D., Busconi, A. & Houchens, P. (1999) 'Developmental and etiological characteristics of children with sexual behaviour problems: treatment implications', *Child Abuse and Neglect*, 23(6): 601–621.

Gray, C. (2000) *The New Social Story Book*. Arlington, TX: Future Horizons.

Green, C. S. & Bavelier, D. (2006) 'Enumeration versus multiple object tracking: the case of action video game players', *Cognition*, 101: 217–245.

Greenberg, M., Howes, F., Waters, E., Maher, E. & Oberklaid, F. (2005) 'Promoting the social and emotional health of primary school-aged children: reviewing the evidence base for school-based interventions', *International Journal of Mental Health Promotion*, 7: 30–36.

Griffiths, L. J., Hawkins, S. S., Cole, T. J. & Dezateux, C. (2010) 'Risk factors for rapid weight gain in preschool children: findings from a UK-wide prospective study', *International Journal of Obesity*, 34(4): 624–632.

Gunning, N. & Nicholson, S. (2010) 'Drinking alcohol', in E. Fuller & M. Sanders (eds) *Smoking, Drinking and Drug Use Among Young People in England in 2009*. London: NHS Information Centre for Health and Social Care.

Hackett, S. (2011) 'Children and young people with harmful sexual behaviours', in C. Barter & D. Berridge (eds) *Children Behaving Badly: Peer Violence Between Children and Young People*. Chichester: Wiley/Blackwell, pp. 121–135.

Hall, L., Woods, S., Sobral, D., Dautenhahn, K., Paiva, A., Wolke, D. & Newall, L. (2004) 'Designing empathic agents: adults versus kids', in J. C. Lester, R. M. Vicari & F. Paraguaçu (eds) *Proceedings of Intelligent Tutoring Systems 7th International Conference*. Amsterdam: Springer Verlag, pp. 604–613.

Halsey, K., Gulliver, C., Johnson, A., Martin, K. & Kinder, K. (2005) *Evaluation of BESTs*. Slough: NFER.

Harris, P. L. (1989) *Children and Emotion*. Oxford: Basil Blackwell.

Harris, P. L. (1999) 'Acquiring the art of conversation: children's developing conception of their conversation partner', in M. Bennett (ed.) *Developmental Psychology: Achievements and Prospects*. Philadelphia, PA: Psychology Press.

Harris, P. L. (2000) *The World of the Imagination*. Oxford: Basil Blackwell.

Hart, B. & Risley, T. (1995) *Meaningful Differences in Everyday Parenting and Intellectual Development in Young American Children*. Baltimore, MD: Brookes.

Harter, S. (1985) *Self Perception Profile for Children*. Denver, CO: University of Denver Press.

Harter, S. (1993) 'Causes and consequences of low self-esteem in children and adolescents: a meta-analytic review', *Journal of Clinical Child Psychology*, 27: 423–433.

Harter, S. (1999) *The Construction of the Self: A Developmental Perspective*. New York: Guilford Press.

Harwood, R. L., Miller, J. G. & Irizarry, N. L. (1995) *Culture and Attachment: Perceptions of the Child in Context*. New York: Guilford Press.

Haviland, J. M. & Lelwica, M. (1987) 'The induced affect response: 10-week-old infants' responses to three emotion expressions', *Developmental Psychology*, 23: 97–104.

Hawker, D. S. J. & Boulton, M. J. (2000) 'Twenty years' research on peer victimization and psychosocial maladjustment: a meta-analytic review of cross-sectional studies', *Journal of Child Psychology and Psychiatry*, 41(4): 441–455.

Hazan, C. & Zeifman, D. (1994) 'Sex and the psychological tether', in K. Bartholomew & D. Perlman (eds) *Advances in Personal Relationships*. London: Jessica Kingsley.

Ho, Y., Cheung, M. & Chan, A. (2003) 'Music training improves verbal but not visual memory: cross-sectional and longitudinal explorations in children', *Neuropsychology*, 17(3): 439–450.

Hoff, E. (2006) 'How social contexts support and shape language development', *Developmental Review*, 26(1): 55–88.

Hoff, E. (2010) 'Context effects on young children's language use: the influence of conversational setting and partner', *First Language*, 30(3–4): 461–472.

Hoffman, M. (2000) *Empathy and Moral Development: Implications for Caring and Justice.* New York: Cambridge University Press.

Hornsby, B. & Shear, F. (1993) *Alpha to Omega*, 4th edition. Oxford: Heinemann Educational.

Huesmann, L. R. (2007) 'The impact of electronic media violence: scientific theory and research', *Journal of Adolescent Health*, 41: S6–S13.

Humphrey, N., Lendrum, A. & Wigelsworth, M. (2010) *Social and Emotional Aspects of Learning (SEAL) Programme in Secondary Schools: National Evaluation.* Research Report DFE-RR049. London: Department for Education Publications.

Humphrey, N., Kalambouka, A., Bolton, J., Lendrum, A., Wigelsworth, M., Lennie, C. & Farrell, P. (2008) *Primary Social and Emotional Aspects of Learning: Evaluation of Small Group Work.* Research Report RR064, Nottingham: DCSF Publications.

Hurtado, N., Marchman, V. A. & Fernald, A. (2008) 'Does input influence uptake? Links between maternal talk, processing speed and vocabulary size in Spanish-learning children', *Developmental Science*, 11(6): 31–39.

Hyter, Y. & Westby, C. (1996). 'Using oral narratives to assess communicative competence', in A. Kamhi, K. Pollack & J. Harris (eds) *Communication Development and Disorders in African American Children and Youth.* Baltimore, MD: Brookes, pp. 246–266.

Institute of Alcohol Studies (2009) *Adolescents and Alcohol: Problems Related to Drinking.* Accessed August 2011 from www.ias.org.uk/resources/factsheets/adolescents_problems.pdf

Ireson, J. (2000) 'Activity and interaction in pedagogical contexts', in H. Cowie & G. van der Aalsvoort (eds) *Social Interaction in Learning and Instruction.* Amsterdam: Pergamon Press, pp. 129–143.

Jennifer, D. & Williams, S. (2011) *Linking Lies*, London: Lewisham College. Accessed August 2011 from www.lsis.org.uk

Johnson, T. C. & Doonan, R. (2005) 'Children with sexual behaviour problems: what we have learned in the past two decades', in M. C. Calder (ed.) *Children and Young People Who Sexually Abuse: New Theory, Research and Practice.* Lyme Regis: Russell House Publishing.

Joliffe, W. (2004) 'The National Literacy Strategy: not prescriptive enough?' Paper presented at the British Educational Research Association Annual Conference, University of Manchester, 16–18 September.

Jones, S. E., Manstead, A. S. R. & Livingstone, A. G. (2011) 'Ganging up or sticking together? Group processes and children's responses to text-message bullying', *British Journal of Psychology*, 20(1): 71–96.

Kamerman, S. B. & Kahn, A. J. (2004) 'Early Head Start, child care, family support, and family policy', in E. Zigler & S. Styfco (eds) *The Head Start Debates.* Baltimore, MD: Brookes, pp. 415–422.

Karagiannakis, A. & Sladeczek, I. (2009) 'Classwide peer tutoring and students with SEBD', in C. Cefai & P. Cooper (eds) *Promoting Emotional Education*, London: Jessica Kingsley, pp. 93–108.

Keel, P. K. & Brown, T. A. (2010) 'Update on course and outcome in eating disorders', *International Journal of Eating Disorders*, 43: 195–204.

Keel, P. K., Baxter, M. G., Heatherton, T. F. & Joiner, T. E. (2007) 'A 20-year longitudinal study of body weight, dieting, and eating disorder symptoms', *Journal of Abnormal Psychology*, 116: 422–432.

Kermoian, R. & Leiderman, P. H. (1986) 'Infant attachment in mother and child caretaker in an East African community', *International Journal of Behavioral Development*, 9: 455–469.

Kershaw, C., Nicholas, S. & Walker, A. (2008) 'Crime in England and Wales 2007/08', Home Office Statistical Bulletin 07/08. London: Home Office.

Killen, M. & Stangor, C. (2001) 'Children's social reasoning about inclusion and exclusion in gender and race peer group contexts', *Child Development*, 72: 174–186.

Kitzmann, K. M., Cohen, C. & Lockwood, R. L. (2002) 'Are only children missing out? Comparison of the peer-related social competence of only children and siblings', *Journal of Social and Personal Relationships*, 19: 299–316.

Kochanska, G. (2001) 'Emotional development in children with different attachment histories: the first three years', *Child Development*, 72: 474–490.

Kroger, J. (ed.) (2004) *Discussions on Ego-identity*. Hillsdale, NJ: Lawrence Elrbaum.

Kröger, S. (2010) 'Shared experience', *YoungMinds Magazine*, 107: 30–31.

Lazar, I. & Darlington, R. (1982) 'Lasting effects of early education: a report from the Consortium for Longitudinal Studies', *Monographs of the Society for Research in Child Development*, 47(2–3), Series No. 195.

Leach, P., Barnes, J., Malinberg, L.-E., Sylva, K. & Stein, A. (2008) 'The quality of different types of child care at 10 and 18 months: a comparison between types and factors related to quality', *Early Child Development and Care*, 178(2): 33.

Lefkowitz, M. M., Eron, L. D., Walder, L. O. & Huesmann, L. R. (1977) *Growing Up to be Violent*. New York and Oxford: Pergamon Press.

Leman, P. J. & Tenenbaum, H. R. (2011) 'Practising gender: children's relationships and the development of gendered behaviour and beliefs', *British Journal of Developmental Psychology*, 29: 153–157.

Lewis, M. & Brooks-Gunn, J. (1979) *Social Cognition and the Acquisition of Self*. New York: Plenum Press.

Livingstone, S., Haddon, L., Gorzig, A. & Olafsson, K. (2010) *Risks and Safety on the Internet*. London: London School of Economics. Accessed August 2011 from www.eukidsonline.net

Mahady Wilton, M. M., Craig, W. & Pepler, D. (2000) 'Emotional regulation and display in classroom victims of bullying: characteristic expressions of affect, coping styles and relevant contextual factors', *Social Development*, 9: 226–245.

Main, M. & Cassidy, J. (1988) 'Categories of response to reunion with the parent at age 6: predictable from infant attachment classification and stable over a 3-month period', *Developmental Psychology*, 24: 415–426.

Main, M. & Hesse, E. (1990) 'The insecure disorganized/disorientated attachment pattern in infancy: precursors and sequelae', in M. Greenberg, D. Cicchetti & E. M.Cummings (eds) *Attachment in the Preschool Years: Theory, Research and Intervention*. Chicago, IL: University of Chicago Press, pp. 161–182.

Main, M. & Solomon, J. (1990) 'Procedures for identifying infants as disorganized/disoriented during the Ainsworth Strange Situation', in M. T. Greenberg, D. Cicchetti & E. M. Cummings (eds) *Attachment in the Preschool Years: Theory, Research and Intervention*. Chicago, IL: University of Chicago Press, pp. 121–160.

Main, M., Kaplan, N. & Cassidy, J. (1985) 'Security in infancy, childhood, and adulthood: a move to the level of representation', in I. Bretherton & E. Waters (eds) *Growing Points of Attachment Theory and Research. Monographs of the Society for Research in Child Development*, 50(1–2, Serial No. 209): 66–104.

Marcia, J. E. (1970) 'Ego identity status: relationship to change in self-esteem, general maladjustment and authoritarianism', *Journal of Personality*, 35: 118–133.

Marcia, J. E. (1993) 'The relational roots of identity', in J. Kroger (ed.) *Discussions on Ego-identity*. Hillsdale, NJ: Lawrence Erlbaum.

Marsh, H. W. & Craven, R. G. (2006) 'Reciprocal effects of self-concept and performance from a multidimensional perspective', *Perspectives on Psychological Sciences*, 1(2): 133–163.

Marsh, J. (2003) '"Teletubbies" and the language and literacy curriculum in the early years', *Televizion Online*, 16: 1–6. Accessed August 2011 from www.br-online.de/jugend/izi/english /e-marsh.htm

Masten, A. S. & Garmezy, N. (1985) 'Risk, vulnerability, and protective factors in developmental psychopathology', in B. Lahey & A. Kazdin (eds) *Advances in Clinical Child Psychology*, Vol. 8. New York: Plenum Press, pp. 1–52.

Matthews, R., Hunter, J. A. & Vuz, J. (1997) 'Juvenile female sexual offenders: clinical characteristics and treatment issues', *Sexual Abuse: A Journal of Research and Treatment*, 9: 187–199.

Mayseless, O. & Scharf, M. (2007) 'Adolescents' attachment representations and their capacity for intimacy in close relationships', *Journal of Research on Adolescence*, 17(1): 23–50.

Mead, G. H. (1934) *Mind, Self and Society from the Standpoint of a Social Behaviorist*. Chicago, IL: University of Chicago Press.

Media Literacy Task Force (2009) *Digital Britain: An Interim Report*. Accessed 20 July 2009 from www.medialiteracy.org

Meins, E., Fernyhough, C., Fradley, E. & Tuckey, M. (2001) 'Rethinking maternal sensitivity: mothers' comments on infants' mental processes predict security of attachment at 12 months', *Journal of Child Psychology and Psychiatry and Allied Disciplines*, 42(5): 637–648.

Meins, E., Fernyhough, C., Johnson, F. & Lidstone, J. (2006) 'Mind-mindedness in children: individual differences in internal-state talk in middle childhood', *British Journal of Developmental Psychology*, 24: 181–196.

Meins, E., Fernyhough, C., Wainwright, R., Das Gupta, M., Fradley, E. & Tuckey, M. (2002) 'Maternal mind-mindedness and attachment security as predictors of theory of mind understanding', *Child Development*, 73: 1715–1726.

Mental Health Foundation (MHF) (1999) *Bright Futures*. London: Mental Health Foundation.

Mithen, S. (2005) *The Singing Neanderthals*. London: Phoenix.

Moffitt, T. E., Arseneault, L., Belsky, D., Dickson, N., Hancox, R. J., Harrington, H., Houts, R., Poulton, R., Roberts, B. W., Ross, S., Sears, M. R., Thomson, M. W. & Caspi, A. (2011) 'A gradient of childhood self-control predicts health, wealth, and public safety', *Proceedings of the National Academy of Sciences*, 108(7): 2693–2698.

Moore, S. & Rosenthal, D. (2006) *Sexuality in Adolescence: Current Trends*. London: Routledge.

Morford, J. P. & Kegl, J. (2000) 'Gestural precursors to linguistic constructs: how input shapes the form of language', in D. McNeill (ed.) *Language and Gesture*. Cambridge: Cambridge University Press.

Moses, L., Baldwin, D. A., Rosicky, J. G. & Tidball, G. (2001) 'Evidence for referential understanding in the emotions domain at twelve and eighteen months', *Child Development*, 72: 718–735.

Mumme, D. L. & Fernald, A. (2003) 'The infant as onlooker: learning from emotional reactions observed in a television scenario', *Child Development*, 74(1): 221–237.

National Child Measurement Programme (NCMP) (2011) http://www.ic.nhs.uk/ncmp

National Institute for Clinical Excellence (NICE) (2004) *Obesity Guidance on Prevention, Identification, Assessment and Management of Overweight and Obesity in Adults and Children*. London: NICE.

National Institute for Clinical Excellence (NICE) (2008) *Emotional Health and Wellbeing in Primary School*. London: NICE.

National Institute for Clinical Excellence (NICE) (2009a) *Emotional Health and Wellbeing in Secondary School.* London: NICE.

National Institute for Clinical Excellence (NICE) (2009b) *Promoting Physical Activity for Children and Young People.* London: NICE.

National Obesity Observatory (NOO) (2009) *Body Mass Index as a Measure of Obesity.* Oxford: National Obesity Observatory.

National Obesity Observatory (NOO) (2011) *Obesity and Ethnicity.* Accessed August 2011 from http://www.noo.org.uk/NOO_pub/briefing_papers

National Treatment Agency for Substance Misuse (2010) *Substance Misuse Among Young People: The Data for 2008–2009.* London: NHS. Accessed April 2011 from http://www.nta.nhs.uk/

Naylor, P. B., Cowie, H., Walter, S. J. & Dawkins, J. (2009) 'Impact of a mental health teaching programme on adolescents', *British Journal of Psychiatry*, 194: 365–370.

Nelson, K. & Fivush, R. (2000) 'Socialization of memory', in E. Tulving & F. I. M. Craik (eds) *Oxford Handbook of Memory.* New York: Oxford University Press.

Newson, E. (1994) 'Video violence and the protection of children', *Journal of Mental Health*, 3: 221–227.

Nielsen, M. & Dissanayake, C. (2000) 'An investigation of pretend play, mental state terms and false belief understanding: in search of a metarepresentational link', *British Journal of Developmental Psychology*, 18: 609–624.

Norwich, B. & Kelly, N. (2004) 'Pupils' views on inclusion: moderate learning difficulties and bullying in mainstream and special schools', *British Educational Research Journal*, 30(1): 43–65.

O'Dea, J. A. (2005) 'Prevention of child obesity: "first, do no harm"', *Health Education Research*, 20(2): 259–265.

Office for National Statistics (ONS) (2011a) *Quality of Ethnicity and Gestation Data Subnationally for Births and Infant Deaths in England and Wales (2005–2008).* London: Office for National Statistics. Accessed August 2011 from www.ons.gov.uk/

Office for National Statistics (ONS) (2011b) *Conceptions in England and Wales 2009.* Accessed August 2011 from http://www.ons.gov.uk/ons/index.html

Office for Standards in Education (OFSTED) (2011) *Supporting Children With Challenging Behaviour Through a Nurture Group Approach.* London: OFSTED, Reference 100230.

Olweus, D. (1993) *Bullying: What We Know and What We Can Do.* Oxford: Basil Blackwell.

Oppenheimer, L. & Barrett, M. (2011) 'National identity and in-group/out-group attitudes in children: the role of sociohistorical settings. An introduction to the special issue', *European Journal of Developmental Psychology*, 8: 1–4.

Papadopoulos, L. (2010) *Sexualisation Review of Young People.* London: Home Office. Accessed August 2011 frm www.homeoffice.gov.uk/documents/Sexualisation-young-people.pdf

Parkes, C. M. (1972) *Bereavement: Studies of Grief in Adult Life.* London: Tavistock.

Paxton, S. J. & Heinicke, B. E. (2008) 'Body image', in S. Wonderlich, J. E. Mitchell, M. de Zwann & H. Steiger (eds) *Annual Review of Eating Disorders Part 2.* Oxford: Radcliffe Publishing, pp. 69–83.

Pempek, T. A. & Calvert, S. (2009) 'Tipping the balance: use of advergames to promote consumption of nutritious foods and beverages by low-income African American children', *Archives of Pediatric Adolescent Medicine*, 163(7): 633–637.

Pepler, D. J. & Craig, W. M. (1998) 'Assessing children's peer relationships', *Child Psychology and Psychiatry Review*, 3: 176–182.

Petrides, K. V. & Furnham, A. (2001) 'Trait emotional intelligence: psychometric investigation with reference to established trait taxonomies', *European Journal of Personality*, 15: 425–448.

Petrides, K. V., Sangareau, Y., Furnham, A. & Frederiskson, N. (2006) 'Trait emotional intelligence and children's peer relations at school', *Social Development*, 3: 537–547.

Physical Education Teachers' Exergaming Resource (2010) *July 9: Teachers Demand Physical Education Overhaul*. Accessed 17 August 2010 from http://www.prlog.org/10776034-teachers-demand-physical-education-overhaul.html

Piaget, J. (1936) *The Origin of Intelligence in the Child*. London: Routledge and Kegan Paul.

Pinker, S. (1994) *The Language Instinct*. London: Allen Lane.

Pinker, S. (2007) *The Stuff of Thought: Language as a Window into Human Nature*. New York: Viking Penguin.

Posada, G., Gao, Y., Wu, F., Posada, R., Tascon, M., Shoelmerich, A., Sagi, A., Kondo-Ikemura, K., Haaland, W. & Synnevaag, B. (1995) 'The secure base phenomenon across cultures: children's behaviour, mothers' preferences, and experts' concepts', in E. Waters, B. E. Vaughn, G. Posada & K. Kondo-Ikemura (eds) *Caregiving, Cultural, and Cognitive Perspectives on Secure-base Behaviour and Working Models: New Growing Points of Attachment Theory and Research. Monographs of the Society for Research in Child Development*, 60(2–3, Serial No. 244): 27–48.

Print, B., Morrison, T. & Henniker, J. (2001) 'An inter-agency assessment framework for young people who sexually abuse: principles, processes and practicalities', in M. C. Calder (ed.) *Juveniles and Children Who Sexually Abuse: Frameworks for Assessment*, 2nd edition. Lyme Regis: Russell House Publishing.

Rait, S., Monsen, J. & Squires, G. (2010) 'Cognitive behaviour therapies and their implications for applied educational psychology', *Educational Psychology in Practice*, 26(2): 105–122.

Ramey, C. T., Campbell, F. A., Burchinal, M., Skinner, M. L., Gardner, D. M. & Ramey, S. L. (2000) 'Persistent effects of early childhood education on high-risk children and their mothers', *Applied Developmental Sciences*, 4(1): 2–14.

Reynolds, S., Mackay, T. & Kearney, M. (2009) 'Nurture Groups: a large scale, controlled study of effects on development and academic attainment', *British Journal of Special Education*, 36(4): 204–212.

Rivers, I. (2011) 'Homophobia and peer violence', in C. Barter & D. Berridge (eds) *Children Behaving Badly: Peer Violence Between Children and Young People*. Chichester: Wiley/Blackwell, pp. 137–151.

Rivers, I. & D'Augelli, A. R. (2001) 'The victimization of lesbian, gay, and bisexual youths: implications for intervention', in A. R. D'Augelli & C. J. Patterson (eds) *Lesbian, Gay and Bisexual Identities and Youth: Psychological Perspectives*. New York: Oxford University Press, pp. 199–223.

Rivers, I. & Gordon, K. (2010) '"Coming out", context, and reason: first disclosure of sexual orientation and its consequences', *Psychology and Sexuality*, 1(1): 21–33.

Rivers, I. & Noret, N. (2010) '"Ih8u": findings from a five-year study of text and e-mail bullying', *British Educational Research Journal*, 36(4): 643–671.

Robbins, C. & Ehri, L. C. (1994) 'Reading storybooks to kindergartners helps them learn new vocabulary words', *Journal of Educational Psychology*, 86(1): 54–64.

Roberts, S. & Howard, S. (2005) 'Watching Teletubbies. Television and its very young audience', in J. Marsh (ed.) *Popular Culture, New Media and Digital Literacy in Early Childhood*. London: Routledge.

Robertson, J. (1971) 'Young children in brief separation – a fresh look', *Psychoanalytic Study of the Child*, 26: 264–315.

Rogers, R. A. (2010) 'Soft benefits for hard nuts: the impact of community-building interventions on "anti-social" youth', *Pastoral Care in Education*, 28(3): 195–204.

Rowe, M. L. & Goldin-Meadow, S. (2009) 'Early gesture selectively predicts later language learning', *Developmental Science*, 12(1): 182–187.

Ruck, M. D., Tenenbaum, H. R. & Sines, J. (2007) 'Brief report: British adolescents' views about the rights of asylum-seeking children', *Journal of Adolescence*, 30: 687–693.

Ruffman, T., Slade, L. & Crowe, E. (2002) 'The relation between children's and mothers' mental state language and theory-of-mind understanding', *Child Development*, 73: 734–751.

Rutter, M. (2000) 'Psychosocial influences: critiques, findings and research needs', *Development and Psychopathology*, 12: 375–405.

Rutter, M. (2007) 'Sure Start Local Programmes: an outsider's perspective', in J. Belsky, J. Barnes & E. Melhuish (eds) *The National Evaluation of Sure Start*. Bristol: The Policy Press, pp. 197–210.

Rutter, M. and the English and Romanian Adoptees (ERA) team (1998) 'Developmental catch-up and deficit following adoption after severe global early privation', *Journal of Child Psychology and Psychiatry*, 39(4): 465–476.

Rutter, M. & Smith, D. J. (1995) (eds) *Psychosocial Disorders in Young People: Time, Trends and their Causes*. Chichester: Wiley.

Rutter, M., Kim-Cohen, J. & Maughan, B. (2006) 'Continuities and discontinuities in psychopathology between childhood and adult life', *Journal of Child Psychology and Psychiatry*, 47(3/4): 276–295.

Rutter, M., Beckett, C., Castle, J., Kreppner, J., Stevens, S. & Sonuga-Barker, E. (2009) *Policy and Practice Implications from the English and Romanian Adoptees (ERA) Study: Forty-five Key Questions*. London: British Association for Adoption and Fostering.

Salmivalli, C. (2010) 'Bullying and the peer group: a review', *Aggression and Violent Behavior*, 36: 81–94.

Salovey, P. & Mayer, J. D. (1990) 'Emotional intelligence', *Imagination, Cognition and Personality*, 9: 185–211.

Samaritans (2000) *Young Men Speak*. Surrey: Samaritans.

Saxton, M. (2010) *Child Language: Acquisition and Development*. London: Sage.

Schieffelin, B. B. & Ochs, E. (1998) 'A cultural perspective on the transition from prelinguistic to linguistic communication', in M. Woodhead, D. Faulkner & K. Littleton (eds) *Cultural Worlds of Early Childhood*. London: Routledge, pp. 48–63.

Schwarz, B. B. & Linchevski, L. (2007) 'The role of task design and argumentation in cognitive development during peer interaction: the case of proportional reasoning', *Learning and Instruction*, 17(5): 510–531.

Scottish Government (2008) *Future Health and Well-being: Healthy Eating, Active Living*. Edinburgh: Scottish Government.

Sear, R. & Mace, R. (2007) 'Who keeps the children alive? A review of the effects of kin on infant survival', *Evolution and Human Behaviour*, 29(1): 1–18.

Senechal, M. (1997) 'The differential effect of storybook reading on preschoolers acquisition of expressive and receptive vocabulary', *Journal of Child Language*, 24: 123–138.

Skiba, R., Reynolds, C. R., Graham, S., Sheras, P., Conoley, J. C. & Garcia-Vazquez, E. (2008) 'Are zero tolerance policies effective in the schools?', *American Psychologist*, 63: 852–862.

Smith, P. K. (2010) *Children and Play*. Chichester: Wiley/Blackwell.

Smith, P. K. (2011) *Bullying. Highlight No. 261*. London: National Children's Bureau.

Smith, P. K. & Cowie, H. (2010) 'Perspectives on emotional labour and bullying: reviewing the role of emotions in nursing and healthcare', *International Journal of Work, Organisation and Emotion*, 3(3): 227–236.

Smith, P. K., Cowie, H. & Blades, M. (2011) *Understanding Children's Development*, 5th Edition. Chichester: Wiley/Blackwell.

Smith, P. K., Mahdavi, J. & Carvallo, M. (2008) 'Cyberbullying: its nature and impact in secondary school pupils', *Journal of Child Psychology and Psychiatry*, 49(4): 376–385.

Smith, P. K., Pepler, D. & Rigby, K. (eds) (2004a) *Bullying in Schools: How Successful Can Schools Be?* Cambridge: Cambridge University Press.

Smith, P. K., Talamelli, L., Cowie, H., Naylor, P. & Chauhan, P. (2004b) 'Profiles of non-victims, escaped victims, continuing victims and new victims in school bullying', *British Journal of Educational Psychology*, 24: 565–581.

Smith, T. & Curran, A. (2010) *Right Time, Right Place: Alcohol-harm Reduction Strategies with Children and Young People*. London: Alcohol Concern.

Snow, P. (2009) 'Oral language competence in childhood and access to equity in education and health across the lifespan', in K. Bryan (ed) *Communication in Healthcare*. Bern: Peter Lang, pp. 101–134.

Snowling, M. J. (2002) 'Reading and other learning difficulties', in M. Rutter & E. Taylor (eds) *Child and Adolescent Psychiatry*, 4th edition. Oxford: Blackwell Scientific, pp. 682–696.

Sourander, A., Brunstein Klomek, A. B., Ikomen, M., Lindroos, J., Luntamo, T., Koskelainen, M., Ristkari, T. & Helenius, H. (2010) 'Psychosocial risk factors associated with cyberbullying among adolescents', *Archives of General Psychiatry*, 67(7): 720–728.

Stanley, N., Ellis, J. & Bell, J. (2011) 'Delivering preventive programmes in schools: identifying gender issues', in C. Barter & D. Berridge (eds) *Children Behaving Badly: Peer Violence Between Children and Young People*. Chichester: Wiley/Blackwell, pp. 217–230.

Starkey, H. (2005) 'Language teaching for democratic citizenship', in A. Osler & H. Starkey (eds) *Citizenship and Language Learning*. London: Sage, pp. 23–39.

Steele, H., Steele, M. & Fonagy, P. (1996) 'Associations among attachment classifications of mothers, fathers and their infants: evidence for a relationship-specific perspective', *Child Development*, 67: 541–555.

Steinberg, L. (2008) *Adolescence*, 8th edition. New York: McGraw-Hill.

Steinberg, L. & Monahan, K. C. (2007) 'Age differences in resistance to peer influence', *Developmental Psychology*, 43: 1531–1543.

Stern, D. (2001) 'Face-to-face play', in J. Jaffe, B. Beebe, S. Feldstein, C. Crown & M. D. Jasnow (eds) *Rhythms of Dialogue in Infancy: Coordinated Timing in Development, Monographs of the Society for Research in Child Development* (Vol. 66). Ann Arbor, MI: SRCD.

Sutton-Smith, B. (2003) 'Play as a parody of emotional vulnerability', in J. Roopmarine (ed.) *Play and Educational Theory and Practice, Play and Culture Studies*. Westport, CT: Praeger.

Sveinson, K. (2008) *A Tale of Two Englands – 'Race' and Violent Crime in the Press*. Accessed August 2011 from http://www.runnymedetrust.org/uploads/publications/pdfs/TwoEnglands-2008.pdf

Swann, W. B., Chang-Schneider, C. & McClarty, K. L. (2007) 'Do people's self-views matter?: self-concept and self-esteem in everyday life', *American Psychologist*, 62(2): 84–94.

Sylva, K., Stein, A. & Leach, P. (2009) 'A prospective study of the effects of different kinds of care on children's development in the first five years', *Families, Children and Child Care Project Report*. London: Tedworth and Glass-House Trusts.

Sylva, K., Melhuish, E., Sammons, P., Siraj-Blatchford, I. & Taggart, B. (2004) *The Effective Provision of Pre-school Education (EPPE) Project: Final Report: A Longitudinal Study Funded by The DfES 1997–2004*. London: DfES.

Sylva, K., Melhuish, E., Sammons, P., Siraj-Blatchford, I., Taggart, B. & Elliott, K. (2003) *The Effective Provision of Pre-school Education (EPPE) Project: Findings from the Pre-school Period*. University of London: Institute of Education.

Takahashi, K. (1986) 'Examining the strange situation procedure with Japanese mothers and 12-month-old infants', *Developmental Psychology*, 22: 265–270.

Takriti, R., Buchanan-Barrow, E. & Barrett, M. (2000) 'Children's perceptions of their own and one other religious group', Poster presented at the XVIth Biennial Meeting of the *International Society for the Study of Behavioural Development Conference*, Beijing, China, July 2000.

Talwar, V. & Lee, K. (2002) 'Development of lying to conceal a transgression: children's control of expressive behaviour during verbal deception', *International Journal of Behavioral Development*, 26(5): 436–444.

Tate, S., Wu, J., McQuaid, J., Cummins, K., Shriver, C., Krenek, M., Brown, S. (2008) 'Comorbidity of substance dependence and depression: role of life stress and self-efficacy in sustaining abstinence', *Psychology of Addictive Behaviors*, 22(1): 47–57.

Tatlow-Golden, M. & Guerin, S. (2010) 'My favourite thing to do and my favourite people: exploring salient aspects of children's self-concept', *Childhood*, 17(4): 545–562.

Taylor, J. F. (2003) 'Children and young people accused of child sexual abuse: a study within a community', *Journal of Sexual Aggression*, 9(1): 57–70.

Testa, A. & Coleman, J. (2006) *Sexual Health Knowledge, Attitudes and Behaviours Among Black and Minority Youth in London*. Brighton: Trust for the Study of Adolescence, and the Naz project. Accessed August 2011 from www.youngpeopleinfocus.org.uk

Tomasello, M. (2003) *Constructing a Language: A Usage-based Theory of Language Acquisition*. Cambridge, MA: Harvard University Press.

Tomasello, M., Akhtar, N., Dodson, K. & Rekau, L. (1997) 'Differential productivity in young children's use of nouns and verbs', *Journal of Child Language*, 24: 373–387.

Tomasello, M., Carpenter, M., Call, J., Behne, T. & Moll, H. (2005) 'Understanding and sharing intentions: the origins of cultural cognition', *Behavioral and Brain Sciences*, 28(5): 675–691.

Toynbee, F. (2009) 'The perspectives of young people with SEBD about educational provision', in C. Cefai & P. Cooper (eds) *Promoting Emotional Education*. London: Jessica Kingsley, pp. 27–56.

Ttofi, M. M. & Farrington, D. P. (2009) *School-based Programs to Reduce Bullying and Victimization. Campbell Systematic Reviews*. Oslo: Campbell Collaboration. Accessed August 2011 from http://www.campbellcollaboration.org/news_/reduction_bullying_schools.php/

UK Internet Security Report (2009) *Get Safe Online: State of the Nation Report*. Accessed August 2011 from www.getsafeonline.org

United Nations (UN) (1989) *Convention on the Rights of the Child*. Geneva: Office of the United Nations High Commissioner for Human Rights. Accessed 9 March 2007 from http://www.unicef.org/crc

United Nations Children's Fund (UNICEF) (2007) *Child Poverty in Perspective: An Overview of Child Well-being in Rich Countries*. Florence: UNICEF Innocenti Research Centre.

United Nations Children's Fund (UNICEF) (2010) *The Children Left Behind: A League Table of Inequality in Child Well-being in the World's Richest Countries*. Innocenti Report Card 9. Florence: UNICEF Innocenti Research Centre.

Van IJzendoorn, M. H. & Kroonenberg, P. M. (1988) 'Cross-cultural patterns of attachment: a meta-analysis of the strange situation', *Child Development*, 59: 147–156.

Van IJzendoorn, M. H. & Sagi, A. (1999) 'Cross-cultural patterns of attachment: universal and contextual dimensions', in J. Cassidy & P. R. Shaver (eds) *Handbook of Attachment*. New York: Guilford Press, pp. 713–734.

Viner, R. M., Cole, T. J., Fry, T., Gupta, S., Kinra, S., McCarthy, D., Saxena, S., Taylor, S.,

Wells, J. C. K., Whincup, P. & Zaman, M. J. S. (2010) 'Insufficient evidence to support separate BMI definitions for obesity in children and adolescents from South Asian ethnic groups in the UK', *International Journal of Obesity*, 34(4): 656–658.

Vydelingum, V. & Colliety, P. (2011) 'The need for a culturally sensitive approach to care', in R. Davies & L. Davies (eds) *Children and Young People's Nursing: Principles for Practice*. London: Hodder Arnold, pp. 57–90.

Vygotsky, L. (1962) *Thought and Language*. Cambridge, MA: MIT Press.

Waller, M. (2010) 'A fixed point in time: bringing the "new" into the primary classroom'. Proceedings of the ESRC Seminar series *Children's and Young People's Digital Literacies in Virtual Online Space*, Seminar 5 – *Virtual Literacies in Schools*, May, Sheffield Hallam University. Accessed August 2011 from www.changinghorizons.net

Watson, S., Vannini, N., Davis, M., Woods, S., Hall, M. and Dautenhahn, K. (2007) *FearNot! An Anti-Bullying Intervention: Evaluation of an Interactive Virtual Learning Environment*, www.e-circus.org

Weare, K. (2004) *Developing the Emotionally Literate School*. London: Paul Chapman.

Webster-Stratton, C., Reid, M. J. & Stoolmiller, M. (2008) 'Preventing conduct problems and improving school readiness: evaluation of the Incredible Years Teacher and Child Training Programs in high-risk schools', *Journal of Child Psychology and Psychiatry*, 49: 471–488.

Wellman, H. M., Baron-Cohen, S., Caswell, R., Gomez, J. C., Swettenham, J., Toye, E. & Lagattuta, K. (2002) 'Thought bubbles help children with autism acquire an alternative to a theory of mind', *Autism*, 6(4): 343–363.

Werner, E. E. & Smith, R. S. (1982) *Vulnerable but Invincible: A Longitudinal Study of Resilient Children and Youth*. New York: McGraw-Hill.

Willoughby, B. L. B., Malik, N. M. & Lindahl, K. M. (2006) 'Parental reactions to their sons' sexual orientation disclosures: the roles of family cohesion, adaptability and parenting style', *Psychology of Men & Masculinity*, 7: 14–26.

Wood, J. & Alleyne, E. (2010) 'Street gang theory and research: where are we now and where do we go from here?', *Aggression and Violent Behaviour*, 15: 100–111.

Woodhead, M. (2009) 'Child development and the development of childhood', in J. Qvortrup, W. Corsaro & M. S. Honig (eds) *The Palgrave Handbook of Childhood Studies*. London: Falmer, pp. 41–61.

Woodhead, M. & Faulkner, D. (2008) 'Subjects, objects or participants? Dilemmas of psychological research with children', in P. Christensen & A. James (eds) *Research With Children*, 2nd edition. London: Routledge, pp. 10–39.

World Health Organization (WHO) (2002) *World Health Report: Reducing Risks, Promoting Healthy Life*. Geneva: WHO.

YoungMinds (2010) *Stigma: A Review of the Evidence*. London: YoungMinds. Accessed August 2011 from www.youngminds.org.uk

Youth Justice Board (2004) *National Evaluation of Restorative Justice in Schools Programme*. London: Youth Justice Board. Accessed August 2011 from www.youth-justice-board.gov.uk

Zigler, E., & Styfco, S. J. (2004) *The Head Start Debates*. Baltimore, MD: Brookes.

Zosuls, K. M., Martin, C. L., Ruble, D. N., Miller, C. F., Gaertner, B. M., England, D. E. & Hill, A. P. (2011) '"It's not that we hate you": understanding children's gender attitudes and expectancies about peer relationships', *British Journal of Developmental Psychology*, 29: 288–304.

Zwaan, M. & Steiger, H. (eds) (2005) *Annual Review of Eating Disorders Part 1*. Oxford: Radcliffe Publishing.

Index

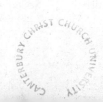